THE
TRULY CURED
CHILD

THE TRULY CURED CHILD

The New Challenge in Pediatric Cancer Care

Edited by
Jan van Eys, M.D., Ph.D.
Head, Department of Pediatrics
University of Texas System Cancer Center
M. D. Anderson Hospital and Tumor Institute

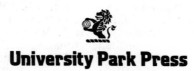

University Park Press

Baltimore · London · Tokyo

Proceedings of a workshop held by the Department of Pediatrics, The University of Texas System Cancer Center, M. D. Anderson Hospital and Tumor Institute, Houston, Texas, on March 13 and 14, 1976.

UNIVERSITY PARK PRESS
International Publishers in Science and Medicine
Chamber of Commerce Building
Baltimore, Maryland 21202

Typeset by The Composing Room of Michigan, Inc.
Manufactured in the United States of America by Universal Lithographers, Inc., and The Optic Bindery Incorporated

Library of Congress Cataloging in Publication Data
Main entry under title:

The truly cured child.

"Proceedings of a workshop held by the Department of Pediatrics, the University of Texas System Cancer Center, M. D. Anderson Hospital and Tumor Institute, Houston, Texas, on March 13 and 14, 1976."
Includes index.
1. Tumors in children—Psychological aspects—Congresses. 2. Children—Hospital care—Moral and religious aspects—Congresses. 3. Pediatrics—Philosophy—Congresses. I. Van Eys, Jan. II. Anderson Hospital and Tumor Institute, Houston, Tex. Dept. of Pediatrics. [DNLM: 1. Neoplasms—In infancy and childhood—Congresses. QZ200 T866 1976]
RC281.C4T78   618.9'29'94   77-416
ISBN 0-8391-1108-8

CONTENTS

CONTRIBUTORS

Richard Benton, Ph.D., Department of Rehabilitation Medicine, Staff Psychologist

George Blumenschein, M.D., Assistant Director of Education

Margaret Buchorn, M.A., Social Psychotherapist

Annabelle Chavez, R.N., Head Nurse, Inpatient Pediatric Service

Joseph O'Donnell, C.S.C., Chaplain, Resident in Medical Ethics

Don Peterson, Parent

Ginger Peterson, R.N., Parent

Lois Poitras, R.N., Pediatric Nurse Supervisor

Ellen Richie, Ph.D., Assistant Professor of Pediatrics and Assistant Immunologist

Terry Rulfs, B.A., Graduate Student in Psychology, Texas A & M University, on Practicum in the Pediatric Service at M. D. Anderson Hospital and Tumor Institute

Warren Rutherford, M.B.A., M.H.A., Associate Administrator

Charles R. Shaw, M.D., Professor of Biology and Associate Professor of Pediatrics in Psychiatry

Jan van Eys, Ph.D., M.D., Professor of Pediatrics and Pediatrician

Kenneth Vaux, Dr. Theol., Professor of Ethics

All the staff of M. D. Anderson Hospital who gave their spare time out of their concern for and dedication to the child with cancer

FOREWORD

Faulty communication often results from different perceptions of a situation. The most frequent consequences of communication breakdown, particularly in a hospital, are reduced performance and less gratification for all concerned—the patient, family members, and members of the health care team; sometimes there is even an effect on response to therapeutic measures.

The presentations and shared perceptions of the participants in the workshop described here, sponsored by the Department of Pediatrics of The University of Texas System Cancer Center, M. D. Anderson Hospital and Tumor Institute, show clearly the urgent need for better performance and understanding through better communication. Gratified persons perform more productively and thereby continually reinforce their ability to contribute and to learn.

We are proud that members of our institution are greatly concerned with ill people, dedicated to the concept of the truly therapeutic community, and willing to reevaluate philosophies and routines and seek better ways to serve, learn, and progress.

Combined efforts such as this workshop, in which patients, parents, clergy, and other members of the health care team participated as concerned equals to find solutions to mutual problems, are essential in specialized institutions such as our cancer center. We congratulate our Department of Pediatrics for organizing this workshop and its subsequent publication, and for promoting the concept of the therapeutic community.

R. Lee Clark

PREFACE

Society's commitment to eliminate cancer as a major cause of morbidity and mortality has borne fruit in at least one area—pediatric oncology, the study of cancer in children. An ongoing survey of newly diagnosed children admitted to M. D. Anderson Hospital and Tumor Institute shows that 51 percent remain well and free of disease for more than five years. Mortality figures for childhood cancer show a significant decrease nationwide. The implications of this progress are enormous. Today cure must be considered the norm rather than the exception. Those of us who treat children with cancer must keep their future, not just their cancer in mind. It is still difficult for oncologists to accept the possibility of cure, and much may still happen to children who have survived their first malignancy, but we must be prepared for success. If a cured child is possible, a *truly cured child* is necessary. Truly cured children are not just biologically cured, free of disease, but developmentally on a par with their peers and at ease with their experience of having had cancer.

To make this conceptual change in the management of our children at M. D. Anderson Hospital and Tumor Institute, we held a workshop for all those involved with the children, including volunteers, laboratory workers, researchers, nurses, social service and chaplaincy service personnel, students, fellows, physicians, parents, and patients. *The Truly Cured Child* is a record of that workshop. Through it, we hope to convey that a therapeutic community should be possible and satisfactory to almost everyone. We also show that it is possible for all to sit down as equals and discuss concerns in a way that is not crisis oriented, but future directed.

The problem of achieving a truly cured child is not unique to cancer care. All potentially life-threatening, chronic diseases of childhood challenge the adult world in the same manner. Therefore, this book could be profitably read by all those who care for children. It should be especially helpful to nurses, chaplaincy service personnel, laboratory workers, and volunteers, all of whom carry such a heavy burden but who are often frustrated because they are not heard when decisions are made. It should be read by parents and patients to show them that their concern for the future can and should be shared by a combined medical staff. It should be of value to students of biomedical ethics, who will see ethical and moral principles applied rather than simply discussed in our workshop. This workshop was different in that all came as equals and all were heard. By offering a look into our community, we hope others will compare it to their own.

A brief introduction to our setting is necessary. M. D. Anderson Hospital and Tumor Institute is part of The University of Texas System Cancer Center, Houston, Texas. It is located in the Texas Medical Center, where a concentration of hospitals, medical schools, and institutes has created an exciting environment of medical and ethical inquiry. M. D. Anderson is dedicated to the care of patients with cancer. It is involved in research, teaching, and patient care. The integration of all three in such a way that the patient is truly benefited is a continuing challenge to all who work here. The Department of Pediatrics bears a relatively small proportion of the patient load, but it operates as a separate unit, with its own clinic and ward as well as departmental staff. At the time of the workshop, our inpatient service on 6 West had 32 beds, which was clearly insufficient for the patient load.

The participation of all personnel in a therapeutic community—not only those who deal directly with the patient with cancer, but also those in research and administrative tasks—is necessary and, as this book shows, is possible. Our Department of Pediatrics has tried to show, through its workshop, how this can be accomplished.

ACKNOWLEDGMENTS

The Pediatric Workshop and this subsequent publication would never have been possible without the enthusiasm with which every participant entered into the project. Therefore it would be unreasonable to single anyone out. However, special thanks must go to Wier Smith, who made the physical arrangements, and to Kenneth Vaux, who guided us through the workshop and helped graciously with the editing of the discussion papers. Of course, the workshop could never have taken place without the understanding cooperation of the leadership of The University of Texas System Cancer Center and the Institute of Religion. We are a long way from realizing our therapeutic community, but the workshop gave us renewed hope that it is achievable.

Pediatrics Looks at Itself: The Beginning

CHAPTER 1

Introduction

JAN VAN EYS

The ability of physicians to cure children with malignant diseases as a matter of course is not far in the future. With that new ability it is essential that we are not only prepared for success but that we are also able to generate an environment in which success is optimized. Cancer centers have been pioneers in the development of innovative and multimodal therapy for malignant diseases. It is, therefore, only natural that the centers should be the pioneers in the effective cure of patients with malignant diseases. They must be the vanguard in the restoration of patients to true health.

Because treatment success has been the greatest in childhood tumors, the pediatric services should be the model for the new generation of cancer cure. There is a great interest nationwide in the mental health of the cancer patient and his family.* To make mental health efforts truly successful, however, it is insufficient to graft them onto existing medical programs. Such efforts must be an integral part of the care of the patient and his family from the very beginning.

At M. D. Anderson Hospital and Tumor Institute the Department of Pediatrics struggled for many years with the engraftment approach. The patients benefited greatly from the extra efforts that were put into their care by the mental health team. Physicians learned to use the expertise various members of the team had to offer to the overall management of the patient. This program could be called innovative and successful without being untruthful. It was a team effort, but it was rarely integrated care in the sense that everyone felt equally responsible for the outcome. In fact, the optimal outcome was defined differently by different participants in the care of the children. This problem was not unique to M. D. Anderson Hospital, or to cancer care. The ways in which medical personnel look at patients are so different that often little true communication is possible. Yet this assertion would be vigorously denied by all who do not take time to examine it dispassionately.

An example might be given here which is not from an oncology service and which, therefore, is nonchallenging to those among us who presume our brand of care is optimal. It concerns a large birth-defect service, including neurosurgeons, urologists, pediatricians, orthopedic surgeons, physical therapists, and social workers, with exemplary team

---

*Gender-specific pronouns and adjectives are used throughout this book for convenience. They are not meant to be exclusionary.

effort. All were dedicated to the optimal rehabilitation of severely afflicted children. When a high incidence of anemia was noted, an investigation was launched into its causes. The anemia occurred in almost all the children, most of whom had regular and intensive medical attention. It was not found at the time of initial presentation to the service but developed during the prolonged care. It soon became clear that the anemia was the consequence of blood loss during operations. But the striking fact was that it had been allowed to develop in child after child without any reaction from the house officers because abnormal laboratory values were interpreted as not being unexpected for such abnormal children and therefore not considered to require medical action. Even though there was no reason to relate the anemia to the birth-defect syndrome, the house officers interpreted it in light of their overall impression of the children: "You don't expect them to be normal."[1] This example brings forcibly home the realization that we treat children differently depending on our concepts of them. Since our concepts are as varied as our backgrounds and training, it is evident that our inability to truly communicate lies in part in the fact that we expect different end points for the patients.

We in the Department of Pediatrics at M. D. Anderson Hospital decided that it was necessary to discuss among ourselves our attitudes and concepts, as well as our hopes and expectations. Unlike the usual workshop in which self-satisfied experts show the world how to do their thing, this workshop was designed to summarize the expected and unexpected areas of conflict, as well as the means by which a common purpose could be generated.

Such a common purpose is, of course, the cured child, but even this obvious end point is a semantic morass if not carefully examined. It includes a satisfied family, but the hopes and expectations of families are hardly ever considered concretely because our own values clearly influence the mental image we conjure up of the family with a cured child. It also includes job satisfaction, but that ranges from pride in a successful research career to self-satisfaction generated by patient gratitude. Finally, the common purpose includes a working environment that allows a healthy personal life, unencumbered by unreasonable mental and physical demands.

Because there is a certain degree of uniformity within each subgroup of the care team, many of these points are not problems. There may be a wide span in motivation and ambition among the physicians, but they do understand each other. While the laboratory personnel have sufficiently uniform backgrounds so that they too have shared values, their contact with the patients is incidental. It is often close enough for the child to become a real person, but their inability to actively intervene in the child's care makes it impossible for the patient care aspect to become the exclusive motivating force for them. Yet their realization of the important contribution they make to the overall care is urgent enough to generate an entirely different set of conflicts.

This Pediatric Workshop was designed to give everyone an opportunity to discuss the conflicts between their work and their personal lives, and between ambition and patient care demands. Again, such stress is not unique to the cancer field, but the child who might die generates an overall personal involvement which cannot be ignored and which influences all personal decisions.

We decided to publish the results of this workshop for two reasons. The first was that the experience of such discussions fades very rapidly. Publication would make it possible for the participants to truly remember what was said, and why it was said.

A second reason was that these problems are not limited to our institution. Every large institution tends to lose its coherence and thereby its ability to have a common purpose. Usually this is combated by house organs which describe the virtues of the common goal. Such publishing efforts are liberally sprinkled with praise for the dedicated, for institutions depend on the dedication and the loyalty of individual employees. But if an institution is a patient-care establishment, the patient's welfare may cease to be the common goal of the institution. This does not mean that the patient does not get optimal physical care—quite the contrary. Many conflicts are generated by the need to bring all of the institution's potential to bear on every patient. But conflicts are generated. This workshop, in a sense, was antithetical to the usual house organ in that it resulted in some washing of dirty linen in public. The emphasis, however, was not upon the degree of soiling, but rather upon cleansing the linen through a group discussion, among equals, of common problems. It was not easy to convince all members of the initial planning team that such discussion was possible. Knowledge is only too often equated with importance in care, and stature is frequently confused with humanity.

In this publication of the workshop's proceedings, the discussions have been summarized to produce coherent papers. This was done to highlight the many constructive thoughts of the groups that would have been lost in a verbatim transcript. Many times several themes were developed simultaneously, and many times the vocabulary and the absence of visual support might result in the reader's underestimating the content of the thoughts. Yet in the setting of the discussion group nothing was lost on the participants. There are references to locales known to all participants but without immediate reference to the reader. They have been left because, in context, there is no danger of misunderstanding.

I fervently hope that others may profit from our experience. Our aim was not the democratizing of our care, though if that were a result it would have been beneficial in our eyes. The aim was rather to reach a better understanding of each other in the area of our common task: the care and cure of the child with cancer.

REFERENCE

1. van Eys, J. Normal hematological values in the pediatric age group. Unpublished data, presented as a paper during the symposium, Normal Values in Laboratory Medicine, held May 15–16, 1969, at Vanderbilt University, Nashville, Tenn.

CHAPTER 2

Life-threatening Disease in Children:
The Challenge to Personal and Institutional Values

KENNETH VAUX

My responsibility was to introduce the theme of our conference and to charge our gathering with its task. First I commended those who came, for it is above and beyond the call of duty to give up a weekend with the family for any deliberations, however important. Our presence signaled a commitment to the challenges and values we would explore during the next hours. It is not to a department or an institution that we are dedicated. Indeed, we may be jaded and cynical toward state institutions. We may sympathize with the Arts and Sausages Party which recently elected a new president of The University of Texas-Austin student body. He focused his campaign on a pledge to change the inscription on the main building from, "You shall know the truth and the truth shall make you free" to "Money talks," and to change the university's name to "Fat City." We came not to deride the hospital, nor to extol it. We gathered out of devotion to afflicted children and their families. We are dedicated to save their lives, to dignify their suffering, to share their weeping and rejoicing, to ease their anxiety and support their hope.

Indeed, it is to these goals that M. D. Anderson Hospital and our constituent department, Pediatrics, are committed. When all the bureaucracy is unraveled and all the pettiness, presumptions, and jealousies are laid bare, it is this caring, this vision, that makes this program work. When all is said and done, this commitment is behind the state appropriations, the federal grants, and especially the daily affirmation that prompts each of us to get out of bed and come to work.

I am honored to be an affiliated chaplain with the M. D. Anderson Hospital and a consultant in ethics to the Department of Pediatrics. The lessons of life I have learned at this center are among my most cherished possessions. The fact that we could convene such a meeting is an indication that our institution is coming of age. Some of us can remember when it was absolutely *verboten* to discuss many issues. The emotionality accompanying disease, the mental health dimensions, and the ethical and value realities like death and dying were seen as inappropriate themes for discussion.

But we came, called together by our department chairman because of his deep concern. We met with every encouragement of the administration. We hoped not only that our own sensitivities and sensibilities would be heightened and our work together renewed and refreshed, but

13

that we could record our insights in a published document in which others might find profit.

The theme I posed for consideration was that life-threatening disease in children generates value conflicts both in institutions and in individuals—in patients, parents, and helpers. The word "cancer" sends a chill up the spine. It is life threatening, value devastating. Until recent years it ran relentless and unhindered through the bodies of men, women, and children. Sigmund Freud, who after thirty operations on his neck and jaw had his physician ease him into death, called it "the last disease," a scourge that comes from the very roots of our being. The Romans called it Cancer, the Scorpion, the Krebs—a gnawing, devouring decimator of men. However, some have found the disease benign and friendly—a welcome visitation. In my pastoral experience I have known two elderly women who spoke of cancer as their friend; they greeted it as a message from God, a boatman to take them across the deep river from this troubled shore to that home on the other side. But this gentle rationalization seems alien to modern people with more critical faith, certainly when children are involved. The suffering and death of children was enough to cast Dostoevsky into atheistic despair and rebellion. And with him we ask, why? It seems to contradict the notion of a just universe and a benevolent creator.

Our main concern was not with metaphysical and poetic meanings, important though they be to the sense we make of death and illness. We wanted to examine the concrete, day-to-day values that are thrown into conflict. Our concern was to examine the work of the Department of Pediatrics at M. D. Anderson Hospital and Tumor Institute. What, if any, are the value conflicts set in motion when an institute is committed both to research and to patient care; to fight disease and yet be kind and tender to the sick; to adhere to institutional efficiencies and cost benefit analyses and yet meet the peculiar and spontaneous needs of persons; to follow chains of command, lines of authority and responsibility, and yet have the freedom to abandon and abrogate these customs as we temporarily suspend order in favor of human need?

Several dichotomies served our discussion as a lattice, a framework on which to hang our insights. The first is between engagement and withdrawal. By now it is a cliché to say that work in a unit such as ours demands that we repress our feelings in order to protect ourselves. We must withdraw, become calloused and hard, unwilling to empathize, lest we be immobilized by the burden we bear. It is said that we must keep our distance, maintain objectivity. How else can one administer the medications, do the sticking, endure the sickness caused by the treatment, accept failure and defeat? Patients tell us that the sicker they get, the more critical their illness, the more people withdraw. Their circle of friends shrinks to a few. The doctor, nurse, chaplain, social worker, and attendants appear less often for briefer visits; often only the orderly and cleaning women remain. Failing to find the patience and perseverance to be engaged, we become clock punchers.

Sometimes aloofness is rooted in our personality structure. Some of us are cold and distant, afraid of getting too close, getting involved, and becoming vulnerable. Yet even those who are gregarious and sympathetic need to withdraw and rest, to disengage, restore, repair, and mend. How can we structure our work in order to do this? How can we communicate our love if our countenance signals, "Don't touch!"? How can we be more cognizant of the diversity of gifts in the team? We must all be counselors and consolers at one time or another. How can we enhance these skills?

The second dichotomy is between compassion and contempt. It is compassion that brings parents back to the ward to help another family even after the death of their child. Compassion prompts us to draw near in an honest effort to inform and listen to patients, to bear gracefully the anger they throw out of their pain and frustration. This is what really matters in human transactions. The day can be filled with constant irritations, techniques can fail, the battle can even be lost, but as long as trust and compassion abide there will be no bitterness, even in the midst of profound sorrow. And, I might add, no malpractice.

But compassion is very close to contempt. They are two sides of the same coin. Down through the ages man has had compassion and contempt, often commingled, for the sick. All of us can become contemptuous, though often we fail to realize it. Parents for their children, patients for those who attend them. Often contempt is disguised by a facade of long-suffering kindness. I recently worked with a family at another hospital. The elderly widowed mother was sick and her daughter and son-in-law, though resentful of the burden of coming each day and other constrictions, presented a false face. "It's okay, Mom," they said when she said she didn't want to be a burden. "You're important to us, we don't mind." Outside in the halls they would gripe to and at one another. The mother knew they were exhibiting phoney compassion under which was nothing but contempt. One day I advised the couple to release their true feelings to the old lady and they did. "Mom," they said, "this is a pain in the neck. We can't see our kids, we can't do what we want, we are very angry." Suddenly, and rather remarkably, there developed an honest and mutually supportive relationship in which contempt modulated into genuine love and mutuality. The mother was less demanding; the couple was more understanding. How can we recognize the subtleties of our feelings? How can we open avenues of communication to engender that authenticity that alone makes interactions therapeutic?

Third is the dichotomy between personalized interactivity and professional institutionalism. We are always in danger of hiding behind our professional roles and our sick roles. We allow our science or technique to intervene in the relationship. We become the slaves of protocol and regulation to the point that we miss the aim of all protocol and all policy—namely, patient benefit. How can we be professional, responsible, and yet retain a personalized touch and an interdependence by which we call on each other and rely on each other's unique contribution to the total enterprise?

The last dichotomy, the tension that underlies all others, is that between aggressive action and acceptance. Human life is a process in which we continually attempt to alter those conditions that harm us and finally accept the limitations of our powers. One day not long ago, all medicine could do was resign itself to inevitability in the field of pediatric tumors. Then came the treatments for Wilms' tumor, therapies for Hodgkin's disease, significant remissions in leukemia, as so on. We were and still are on the attack. The scientific commitments and the courage of patients and families are among the noblest expressions yet seen of the glory of man. Defeat often comes, but it is defeat only in a superficial sense. Often a battle can be lost and a war won. Faith and hope drive us on. Death does not defeat our caring inquisitiveness and intervention any more than it extinguishes life's enduring value.

How can we maintain a healthy balance between agressive action and acceptance? How can we approach the wisdom of Niebuhr's prayer: "Lord, give the the courage to change the things that can be changed, the grace to accept that which cannot be changed, and the wisdom to know the difference."

Other dichotomies could have been mentioned, such as being straightforward or labyrinthine in introducing protocols to patients, in imparting diagnoses or prognoses, in telling doctors or nurses how we're doing. But it was time for the conference to get to work.

Therefore, my charge to the conference:

Let us examine what makes for a genuine *therapeutic community,* and what are the impediments in the institution, in the department, in ourselves.

Let us examine the manner of our ministrations as a team in the hospital, in the outpatient clinic, in touch with home care.

Finally, let us be down to earth, honest, candid. Let's call them as we see them, tell it like it is. No one will be fired for expressing his feelings; we are on neutral ground with a common goal to look at what we're doing, to shore up our strengths, to locate and alter our weaknesses, so that we might do a better job in this most demanding place where our God at this time would have us work.

The Conflicts Between the Patient and the Demands Imposed by Institution and Research

CHAPTER 3

Introduction

GEORGE BLUMENSCHEIN

Dr. Vaux's introductory comments helped to set the tone and give direction to the conference. The care of any ill person in our society has become a very complex situation, involving a large and multifaceted health care team. Everything that each member of that team does affects the health of the patient in one way or another, and, in turn, the health of the patient probably affects the actions of each of us in the conduct of our delivery of health care. The care of the cancer patient is more complicated than the care of other patients because of two phenomena:

1. Much of what we do in caring for the cancer patient produces more illness or apparent illness than existed before we started treatment.
2. We deal with diseases with, in many instances, a very definite end point—death.

The Pediatric Workshop was an opportunity for all of us to see how each of us affects the health of the cancer patient in the hospital, and possibly how we react to, or how our health is affected by, the illness in the patient.

In the first morning session we heard from two essential members of the health care team, one representing the biomedical research community and the other representing the hospital administration. Dr. Ellen Richie, assistant professor of pediatrics and an immunologist, discussed the question "Biomedical Research: For the Patient or On the Patient?" Mr. Warren Rutherford, associate administrator of M. D. Anderson Hospital and Tumor Institute, discussed the administrator's view of participation in patient care. Often we place the hospital administration in the role of balancing cost and compassion. Superficially, many of us consider these to be opposing objectives. We were pleasantly surprised to find that these goals are more compatible than we believed them to be.

CHAPTER 4

Biomedical Research: For the Patient or On the Patient?

ELLEN RICHIE

The title of this chapter implies a conflict between the conduct of biomedical research and the interests of those patients who participate as subjects. One of the ultimate goals of biomedical research is to enrich our understanding of biological phenomena and to apply this knowledge to the cure and prevention of disease. Although this is highly optimistic, it is certainly not an unrealistic goal. We have only to recall the explosive progress in science within this century which has resulted in significant strides toward improving public health and well-being to realize the benefits that biomedical research imparts to society. From this vantage point, biomedical research functions for the good of society and therefore for the good of the individuals who collectively form society.

We are interested, however, in learning whether biomedical research always functions for the good of the patient whose participation as a subject is essential for the progress of research. Surely it is the hope of every investigator that his work will result in a significant contribution of immediate value to the patients who have cooperated with him in a research project. It is then far easier to self-assuredly proclaim that biomedical research is *for* the patient. Unfortunately, the objectives of biomedical research are often so long-range that it may be years, even decades, before the knowledge obtained from current studies can be applied to relieve individual suffering. The overall research objectives may be still *for* the patient, but it is the abstract, unidentified future patient who will receive the benefits accrued from the participation of the present patient volunteers. Under these circumstances the question of whether clinical research is *on* or *for* the patient is more likely to disturb one's conscience and to demand consideration of a number of subtle and complex issues.

There are three parties whose input determines the extent and conduct of clinical research: the investigator, the subject (often a patient), and society. In general, the overall objectives of these parties are harmonious and mutually reinforceable. However, underlying conflicts and tensions may exist, and we should acknowledge and seek to remedy them so as to preserve and protect the basic rights and interests of each party. In order to resolve these fundamental conflicts, we must focus our attention on the ethical considerations pertinent to biomedical research.

Since conflicts between scientific advancement and protection of the research subject generally involve research dealing with human participants, one may wonder why it is not possible to avoid dissension by utilizing animal models for research purposes. Dr. Henry Beecher has stated a conclusion reached by many investigators, that "animal experimentation tells us much . . . for a definitive treatment; however, human experimentation is indispensable. . . . Many concepts can be discovered and tested in animals; their establishment in man can be effected only by experimentation in man."[1] Furthermore, Dr. Bradford Gray has pointed out: "Ethical problems cannot be evaded even by abolishing human experimentation—which no one seriously proposes—because the failure to pursue knowledge that might benefit mankind might itself be unethical."[2]

Given that research involving human subjects is indispensable, we must then define human experimentation. Irving Ladimer describes it as "deliberately inducing or altering body or mental functions directly or indirectly, in individuals or in groups, primarily for the advances of health, science and human welfare."[3] Dr. R. A. McCance feels that even the most ordinary, routine clinical procedure may fall within the realm of human experimentation, depending upon the mental attitude of the person conducting the procedure.[4] He regards "collecting an extra specimen of urine or taking an extra 5 cc of blood from a vein puncture made purely for established diagnostic or therapeutic purposes" as experimental since these are unnecessary procedures. McCance also states that all experiments involve some degree of risk, even if infinitesimally small.

The concept of risk versus benefit, as well as the principle of informed consent, have been two of the primary issues in the recent surge of attention concerning the ethics of biomedical research involving human subjects. In recent years a substantial body of evidence has accumulated concerning unequivocal ethical violations in the involvement of human subjects in research projects. Dr. H. K. Beecher made quite an impact with the publication of his article in the *New England Journal of Medicine* documenting several examples of human experimentation in which the ethical rights of individual subjects were clearly ignored.[5] In his subsequent book Beecher addressed himself to those critics of his article who implied that the end justifies the means or that the most important goal is the greatest good for the greatest number: "One can only conclude from their clear statements, as well as inferences, that some critics hold that science, nor morality, is the highest value. Without for a single moment holding any belief in anyone's infallibility in any area, I conclude that some of the criticism of the article mentioned is based upon such surprising attitudes that it is evident that the article or one like it was necessary."[1]

Although much of the concern regarding the exploitation of human subjects has resulted from publicized accounts of dramatic and emotionally charged incidents, there is reason to believe that a general lack of concern on the part of many biomedical investigators is not a highly unusual phenomenon. In 1970 Dr. Bernard Barber and his associates undertook a systematic study of expressed ethical standards as well as actual behavioral practices associated with the use of human subjects in biomedical experimentation. The conclusion was reached that "there is inadequate ethical concern among biomedical investigators that is reflected in excessively risky procedures and that better internal and external controls are essential."[6] The results of this study clearly showed that the majority of investigators were regarded as strict in their awareness of the necessity for informed consent, their unwillingness to accept undue risk for subjects in hypothetical research proposals, and their lack of actual participation in research associated with an unfavorable risk-to-benefit ratio. However, a significant minority of investigators manifested a lack of concern and a more permissive attitude toward these issues.

What factors contribute to this ethical deficiency on the part of a significant minority of the investigators? As in any rapidly advancing, highly competitive field, there are both positive and negative pressures that influence the manner in which individuals deal with various issues. Barber pointed to the struggle for scientific recognition as a strong pressure on investigators faced with decisions involving ethical choices. Those who were more permissive tended to place a higher value on the advancement of scientific knowledge than on ethical treatment of the patient. His study also showed that those investigators who were extreme "mass producers," that is, who tended to publish frequently but were cited only infrequently, were more likely to manifest permissive attitudes toward ethical problems. Negative pressures such as lack of adequate formal or informal ethical training and ineffective control exercised by peer review committees also contributed to lack of ethical considerations. Dr. Geoffrey Edsall believes that investigators "absorbed in the rational process may too often be inadequately equipped to perceive the enormous impact of non-rational determinants in the making of individual or social decisions."[7]

Some investigators have suggested that there has been excessive criticism and an unnecessary intrusion of ethics into biomedical research. Some propose that no further truths can be revealed to those in the biomedical profession who simply follow a "homespun philosophy based on integrity, passion, and the Golden Rule." To this Dr. Ingelfinger, editor of the *New England Journal of Medicine,* has answered, "They (ethicists) do not claim to know the truth. But they do know the philosophical tenets that have shaped mankind's thinking about rightness and wrongness. By virtue of their training, experience, and debate, ethicists recognize the extensive ramifications of ethical issues into conceptual territory of which the untrained person is unaware."[8]

Bradford Gray has noted that "the perspective of the research subject has been largely missing from the dialogue on human experimentation."[2] In conducting an in-depth study on various aspects of human experimentation, Gray interviewed several individuals who had been involved (with or without their awareness) as subjects in a research project. In general, he found that these subjects not only demonstrated a fundamental lack of understanding as to the nature of the research itself but also failed to recognize that they had a choice as to whether they would or would not participate in a research project. One factor suggested to explain the failure of many subjects to exercise independent judgment was the possible role confusion between the therapist—patient relationship and the investigator—patient relationship. Whereas a subject may perceive that he has a certain obligation to cooperate in the former relationship, Gray found that the majority did not feel a similar obligation in the latter relationship. Therefore, the subject must first distinguish the role of the individual (investigator as opposed to therapist) requesting his participation in a research project before he can truly and freely volunteer.

There are certain distinctions between the physician—patient relationship and the investigator—patient relationship. It has been pointed out that "the physician *accepts* patients and is concerned mainly with their welfare; the investigator *selects* subjects—problems as well as individuals—and while responsive to the patient's interests, is more concerned with solving the scientific problems."[9] The conflict of interests inherent when a single person is both physician and investigator has prompted the recommendation that the physician and the investigator be different individuals. The physician can then more impartially protect the patient from the zealous enthusiasm of the researcher. Even when the physician must be at the same time the investigator, "the two attitudes should be recognized and pondered."[9]

The investigator who has little or no patient contact is subject to a conflict of interests similar to that involving the physician–investigator. A primary motivation of the nonphysician investigator who embarks on a career in biomedical research is the desire to discover explanations for biological events that may be consistent with, but not directly applicable to, patient therapy. In his pursuit of scientific knowledge, the investigator must retain a sense of balance concerning the interests of science and the interests of the individual. An investigator cannot abrogate his responsibility to maintain an awareness of ethical problems by relying on the physician to safeguard the patient's rights. As Beecher repeatedly stresses, all individuals involved in biomedical research should remember that "science is not the highest value."

Any attempts to justify ethically questionable research by arguing that it is for the good of society run counter to our deeply rooted traditional belief in the sanctity of the individual. Substitution of the common good for the individual good is professed to be the exception rather than the rule in our society. Dr. Hans Jonas asserts, "A healthy society requires moral treatment of individuals," but he also points out that, under certain conditions, the rights of the individual are conceded to those of society as a matter of moral justness, not mere force.[10] He goes on, "But in making that concession, we require a careful clarification of what the needs, interests, and likes of society are, for society—as distinct from any plurality of individuals—is an abstract and as such is subject to our definition, while the individual is the primary concrete, prior to all definitions, and his basic good is more or less known." Thus, while these concessions are sometimes made, they do not nullify the priority of the individual in society. Research which is more likely to benefit society than the individual is not unethical as long as it is conducted in such a manner that the rights and dignity of the individual subjects are not sacrificed.

The concept of statistical morality is pertinent to the theme of the rights of the individual versus the rights of society. Beecher refers to Warren Weaver's description of statistical morality as derived from "the prejudice against even permitting any one known specific individual to sacrifice his life for the common good." And yet Weaver states, "We have to, in a great many circumstances, submit a lot of individuals to a partial risk . . . [and although] the risk is only one in a million, when a million are involved, the man will be dead with our acquiescence. . . . It is a comfort to our conscience that we don't know where it occurred or when it occurred. But that individual is just as dead as though we knew all about it."[11] Edsall illustrates the situation by referring to the risk of vaccine-associated poliomyelitis when the oral polio vaccine was introduced. Although the risk was alarming, it was minor compared to the advantages offered to society by the vaccine.[7] Not every situation is as easily resolved. In fact, Jonas warns that "the appeal to numbers is dangerous. Is the number of those afflicted by a particular disease great enough to warrant violating the interests of the non-afflicted? Since the number of the latter is usually so much greater, the argument can actually turn around to the contention that the cumulative weight of interest is on *their* side."[10]

In biomedical research there is always the possibility that an experimental protocol will prove detrimental to a few individuals even though a great many more will benefit from the same procedure. The fact that this situation is accepted as an unavoidable consequence of biomedical research may be a reflection of statistical morality. Nevertheless, the concept of statistical morality should not be used as an excuse to disregard the rights of those subjects involved in human experimentation.

Certainly the ethical priorities in every question of individual risk versus public benefit must revolve around the particular issues in the situation at hand. Dr. Joseph Fletcher, author of *Situation Ethics,* has declared, "The core of the ethic . . . is a healthy and primary awareness that 'circumstances alter cases'—i.e., that in actual problems of conscience the situational variables are to be weighed as heavily as the normative or 'general' constants."[12] Situation ethics does not excuse the requirement for a careful application of ethical principles to each unique situation.

Every potential research subject has the right to determine whether the risk to *him* is worth the benefit to *him* or to mankind. The investigator does not have the right to make that decision for the subject. It is incumbent on each investigator to be certain that the subject is aware that he has a choice and can refuse to participate in a research project.

In this regard, a brief comment on the provocative subject of informed consent seems appropriate. The desirability of securing agreement to participate from a truly informed and comprehending subject is a generally agreed upon principle. Each individual has a right, but not a duty, to participate as a subject in biomedical research. Jonas emphasizes that "we must look outside the sphere of the social contact, outside the whole realm of public rights and duties," for motivations that persuade individuals to participate as subjects in research, motivations that society may draw upon but cannot command.[10]

It is also a generally held conviction that truly informed consent is very difficult to achieve for a number of reasons. Frankel has questioned whether the concept of voluntary consent can apply equally to healthy and ill subjects: "Consent does not mean the same thing to a person under the physical and psychological strain of a serious illness as it does to the healthy subject."[13] Gray emphasizes that obtaining informed consent must be an active procedure initiated by the investigator because subjects do not always comprehend the necessity to exercise their own judgment.[2] Too often, he found, subjects cooperate simply because they feel that their physician would not have offered the option were it not to their benefit. Even when a subject volunteers completely of his own free will, it may be difficult to truly inform him of the risks and benefits of an untried drug or procedure. The investigator himself is not absolutely sure of the answers or else he would not be conducting the experiment. Equally important is the fact that the subject cannot be expected to evaluate risks with the same insight as the trained professional.

Because of the complexities inherent in obtaining informed consent, Beecher has repeatedly stressed that, even though difficult, it is a goal toward which we must strive. The resolution of this problem becomes even more precarious when dealing with special groups such as prisoners, the mentally ill, and children. Beecher's guidelines concerning biomedical research involving children are relatively straightforward. First, he believes that there is no need to limit research involving healthy normal children to studies directly beneficial, as long as valid consent from parents or guardians has been obtained, there is no discernible risk, and the research proposal has been carefully reviewed by a high level review committee. In addition, if the child is capable of understanding the situation, his consent should be obtained and his participation should never be forced, even though permission is given by "overzealous or unstable parents or guardians." Children should not be involved as subjects of a research project which entails discernible risk unless it is for their direct benefit. The same general principles would apply for research concerning sick children.

While these guidelines are a useful frame of reference, there are a number of complex ethical issues concerning the participation of children that are not easily categorized into distinct ethical departments. In a provocative article concerning the medical ethics of bone marrow transplantation in children, Levine et al. question whether a child can give a truly informed consent to donate bone marrow to a sibling. They explain, "In asking a child to consent to a procedure, one recognizes his right to significant decision-making power. But implicit in the application of this rightful claim must be the finding that the child has the capacity to represent his own interests. The challenge is to determine when a child is cognitively, morally, and emotionally competent to provide truly informed consent or refusal for such a procedure."[14] The complexity of the competence issue is further illustrated by the hypothetical situation in which a child refuses to provide bone marrow (a procedure of only minimal risk) to a dying sibling. "If this does occur, one will have to face the issue of whether a family or society has the authority to require a child's participation in a medical procedure which is not of any direct benefit to him and which is contrary to his expressed will."[14]

In discussing the issue of informed consent in children, Campbell asserts that "parental permission coupled with the integrity of the investigator must remain the basis for all actions to protect the individual child against unworthy research."[15] These safeguards, together with the protective role of the law, have traditionally served "to protect children from their own incompetence." But, as Levine et al. point out, this viewpoint is now coming under careful scrutiny: "It is clear that we are living in an era of heightened sensitivity to the rights of children. The challenge to pediatricians is to acknowledge and preserve these rights without impeding the advancement and application of modern pediatrics."[14]

The issue of individual versus societal rights converges in the classical conflict of the end versus the means. It is a widely held but not universal conviction that the end cannot justify the means. Beecher asserts, "If a study is unethical, it does not become ethical because it produces useful results."[1] Gross neglect of ethical considerations has occurred when highly admirable research objectives were sought at the expense of individual rights and dignity. Both the end *and* the means are relevant in justifying involvement of human subjects in biomedical research. Even though the end does not justify the means, the end must do justice to the means. As Frankel explains, "In any type of human experimentation, . . . whether it involves patients or healthy volunteers, attempts to balance risks and benefits in order to obtain valid consent become meaningless if the research question is trivial, the experimental design poorly constructed, or the investigator incompetent. It is certainly unethical to ask a subject to assume any risk to obtain information that is trivial or the result of a poorly constructed research design."[13]

To return to the focal issue of this discussion—whether biomedical research is on or for the individual—it seems that each case must be decided on its own merit. Perhaps, however, a few generalizations can be advanced. If a research project is conducted either by means that abuse the rights of the subject or for an end that is trivial, then this research is *on* rather than *for* the patient. If a research project is conducted, as we hope most are, by ethically acceptable means and for a relevant end, then it is not *on* the patient. When the results have direct benefit to the patient, one may presume that it is *for* that patient. On the other hand, if the results are not directly applicable to that patient, then although the research is not *on,* it is still not *for,* the patient. However, in this case the research may be ethically irreproachable on the basis of its potential value for future patients.

Of course, the ethical issues encountered in biomedical research are much more complicated than this highly simplistic evaluation suggests. The terms "ethically acceptable means" and "relevant end" are subject to various interpretations. Gray has commented on the subjectivity involved in applying generally agreed upon principles to specific cases.[2] He has pointed out that, although an acceptable risk-to-benefit ratio is generally acknowledged to be a necessary prerequisite for biomedical research, it is doubtful that all investigators will agree just how low this ratio must be in any given situation. The evolution of biomedical ethics will continue as long as new frontiers are created by biomedical research. Dr. David Callahan feels that wisdom can be gained only by pooling the intellectual resources and experience of both the biomedical investigator and the philosopher. He concludes, "There is nothing harder than distinguishing 'right' from 'wrong,' 'good' from 'bad,' 'better' from worse,' but nothing is so imperative as to make the attempt, just as all other generations have had to do."[16]

REFERENCES

1. Beecher, H. K.: Research and the Individual. Little, Brown, Boston, 1970.
2. Gray, B.: Human Subjects in Medical Experimentation. John Wiley & Sons, New York, 1975.
3. Ladimer, I.: Ethical and legal aspects of medical research on human beings. J. Public Law 3:467, 1954.
4. McCance, R. A.: The practice of experimental medicine. Proc. R. Soc. Med. 44:189. 1951.
5. Beecher, H. K.: Ethics and clinical research. New Engl. J. Med. 274:1354, 1966.
6. Barber, B.: Research on Human Subjects. Russell Sage Foundation, New York, 1973.
7. Edsall, G.: A positive approach to the problem of human experimentation. Daedalus 98:463, 1969.
8. Ingelfinger, F. J.: Ethics and high blood pressure. New Engl. J. Med. 292:43, 1975.
9. Ladimer, I.: Human experimentation: medicolegal aspects. New Engl. J. Med. 257:18, 1957. Paraphrased in Beecher (1).
10. Jonas, H.: Philosophical reflections on experimenting with human subjects. Daedalus 98:219, 1969.
11. Weaver, W.: Comment on the problem of statistical morality. Dartmouth Alumni Mag. (Suppl.): 4, Nov. 1960. Quoted in Beecher (1).
12. Fletcher, J.: Situation Ethics. The Westminister Press, Philadelphia, 1966.
13. Frankel, M.: The development of policy guidelines governing human experimentation of the United States: a case study of public policy-making for science and technology. Ethics Sci. Med. 2:43, 1975.
14. Levine, M. D., Camitta, B. M., Nathan, D., and Curran, W. J.: The medical ethics of bone marrow transplantation in childhood. J. Pediatr. 86:145, 1975.
15. Campbell, A. G. M.: Infants, children and informed consent. Br. Med. J. 3:334, 1974.
16. Callahan, D.: To confront ethical issues in medicine. New Engl. J. Med. 292:315, 1975.

CHAPTER 5

The Institutional Organization: Self-serving or Patient-serving?

WARREN L. RUTHERFORD

Increasing attention and concern are being directed at organizations characterized by their employees, clientele, or the public as "self-serving." In the public service area, utility companies and government agencies have drawn criticism for their lack of concern for those they serve, for looking instead to growth for growth's sake, to maximizing profit, or to maintaining a strong operating position. It is, therefore, not surprising that the hospital or health care institution is suspect and must periodically reevaluate its motives, even its justification for existence, and redirect its efforts to ensure it is truly patient-serving.

In the hospital industry major changes have been made during the past decade. Technological advancements in both diagnostic and treatment phases of health care have brought not only new procedures but a growing number of specialty disciplines and, in turn, specialists whose knowledge is essential to the effective implementation of the new technology. The results, a more complex working environment and more persons of significantly varied backgrounds and concern for patients, interface in direct patient care. In addition, the typical hospital is larger now and prone to such patient criticism as, "They don't know me," and, "No one there really cares." Certainly, through efforts to maximize the cost effectiveness of large-scale equipment and to justify the provision of specialized medical and technical staffs, hospitals have been forced into constant expansion.

It would be inappropriate in a discussion of this nature not to mention increasingly restrictive sources of operating income for hospitals and the passage of an increasing number of laws and regulations constraining the action of health care institutions and necessitating increased control over operations. These developments tend to make more impersonal the relationship of hospitals to patients and also to preclude timely establishment of new services in response to changing needs.

While space will not permit a comprehensive evaluation of these and other factors which might lead to the conclusion that health care institutions are self-serving, it is quite clear hospitals contain many of the elements which might provoke such allegations. It is important, therefore, to evaluate elements in the organization and operation of hospitals that arouse concern as to their true patient-serving qualities.

DISTINCTION BETWEEN PUBLIC SERVICE
AND PROFIT-MAKING ORGANIZATIONS

The subtitle of this chapter cautions us to make a distinction between the public service, institutional type of organization and the typical profit-making business. The distinction I wish to make does not relate to their manner of operation, as I would like to assume agreement that a public service organization must operate in a reasonably businesslike manner if it is to survive and merit the confidence of those it serves. It is rather in terms of the organization's ultimate objective, or the basis on which its effectiveness is to be appraised. Both types of organizations must create customer satisfaction in order to stay in business. But in the case of the profit-making business enterprise, the degree of customer satisfaction is ultimately restricted by the rate of return on capital, or the organization's profit motivation. A public service institution, on the other hand, has as its ultimate purpose maximization of customer satisfaction in the form of service, within the restriction of available capital. Obviously it is contradictory for a public service organization to be self-serving. If it were, it would not be fulfilling the purpose for which it was established.

MANAGEMENT FUNCTIONS OF ALL
INSTITUTIONS ARE BASICALLY SIMILAR

Certain basic business functions are necessary to the survival of all organizations. Peter Drucker says, "The manager in the public service institution faces the same tasks as the manager in a business: to perform the function for the sake of which the institution exists, to make work productive and the worker achieving, to manage the institution's social impacts, and to discharge its social responsibilities."[1] Further, he states, "Public service institutions equally face the challenge of innovation, and have to manage growth, diversity, and complexity." The ultimate goal of every organization should be to maximize performance so as to accomplish a predetermined objective, using most effectively the resources of personnel, time, and money.

It must be recognized in this regard that all organizations function with various restrictions. Many of these ultimately relate to funding or financial resources, but, as mentioned earlier, there are always legal restrictions and governmental regulations to be observed. In the final analysis it is a question of balance—expenditures to income, relative needs between departments or functions, and the allocation of resources in such a manner as to maximize achievable results. The mechanism whereby these functions are accomplished can be described as "management." But a primary responsibility of management is to keep an institution true to its original purpose. In a hospital, this includes maximizing the hospital's public service, patient-serving role and thereby avoiding activities which might be characterized as self-serving.

ORGANIZATIONAL ELEMENTS
FOSTERING SELF-SERVING CONCERNS

Before identifying those elements in a hospital which might be so abused as to foster institutional self-serving concerns, we must first define the term "self-serving." For purposes of this discussion, a self-serving public institution shall be considered one that acts primarily for its own benefit or to satisfy its own internal operational requirements, with little regard for its basic reason for being—public service. In reality, however, we are dealing with degrees, not extremes, of emphasis. An institutional self-serving act may be no more than an unwillingness to disrupt established policy to meet an unusual patient need. In so doing, the institution places its interests over the immediate requirements of one patient. Although we would not condone such an action, we must acknowledge that a degree of self-interest is essential to an organization.

I have indicated that an institution has certain functions it must fulfill if it is to remain in business. George Wren, in discussing the process of management, includes the basic functions of planning, organizing, actuating, and controlling.[2] In order to perform these functions it is necessary for an institution to develop an organizational structure, to delegate responsibility, to develop overall goals and operational objectives, and, through the development of policy and procedures, to set forth guidelines along which the institution is expected to operate. These activities are essential to the organization's survival and to its ability to be patient-serving. It is only when, in the process of fulfilling these functions, an organization places primary emphasis in decision making on its self-perpetuation or on the smoothness of its internal operation, to the detriment of its patient care program, that we have the beginning of a self-serving environment. In such an environment the patient may not be afforded timely intervention in emerging health-related problems or the minimally essential range of life-saving or support services, such as the individual attention and concern he and his family require during periods of stress associated with medical problems. Therefore, as earlier stated, it is a question of degree, a question of emphasis. In a patient-serving institution the pivotal factor to be given consideration in any decision should be the effect on the patient.

EXAMPLES OF SELF-SERVING
RESTRICTIONS ON PATIENT CARE

In attempting to cite examples of organizational elements of a self-serving nature, we must realize that there is no one element which always is self-serving by nature. As we increase the size of an organization, it tends to become more impersonal and personnel are further removed from persons of ultimate authority, necessitating the establishment of more comprehensive guidelines in the form of written policies and procedures. Flexibility in response to specific problems becomes more difficult to maintain.

Procedures for procedures' sake: this is perhaps the principal element of concern in a self-serving institution. However, in a patient-serving environment policies and procedures can be interpreted so as to take into consideration the individual circumstances and needs of the situation. Some policies must be enforced to the letter, but the majority should leave room for interpretation and certainly not be ends in themselves. Policies and procedures should be means to an ideal end of better patient care.

The saying, "Policies are meant to be broken," has validity in a patient-serving organization. But they must be broken with caution and by individuals with appropriate experience and training. Concern must be given to the institution's organizational structure. Without a proper and clear plan of organization, a defined relationship between departments, employees, and supervisors, and the appropriate delegation of authority and responsibility, all too often policies and procedures become unduly restrictive. Wren says, "Decision making can and should be delegated. As a matter of fact, it should be delegated down the organizational line into the lowest competent level. The lowest competent level in the organization is where the decision maker can see the effect of that decision on the total organization."[2] I would add that it should also be where the decision maker can best interpret, in combination, the immediate needs and circumstances of the situation. Written policies and procedures are essential to any organization to assure uniform action and communicate the plans by which patient care services can be most efficiently and effectively provided. But they are made more effective through timely interpretation by properly selected individuals at appropriate levels of the organization.

Let me ask you a question. In selecting a time to schedule a patient test, or serve a patient meal, or draw blood, do we first consider the effect on the patient, or do we consider the effect on the schedules in our department or on the ordinary schedule of activities in the nursing unit? If we are honest with each other, I would imagine there are all too many occasions when we consider first our schedule, to the inconvenience of the patient. Is this not a self-serving operational element? We have heard much about the dehumanizing experience of hospitalization and often we forget that patients have individual tastes and interests. Unfortunately many of our services and procedures are provided on the basis of departmental expediency, without full consideration for patients' immediate needs, expectations, or habits.

A condition characterized by the phrase "too much organization" or "inadequate communication" may work to the detriment of a developing patient care program. Communication is essential to accommodate changing situations and to permit the coordination of individual effort. Conditions requiring potential changes in policy must be communicated if they are to receive proper attention and evaluation. Operating problems must be described and their magnitude must be assessed if they are to be resolved. Sometimes the significance of the variation in policy requires communication prior to action. Other times circumstances will not permit delay or a decision is unlikely to have a harmful effect. At these times a decision should not be delayed, but made in the best interest of the patient, based upon the best information available. Communication can follow and, in most situations, corrective action can be taken to negate any ill effects resulting from the earlier decision.

All too often there tends to be excessive study, review, and evaluation at multiple levels of large organizations. This situation may restrict timely response to problems as they develop and delay the initiation of new programs which may benefit the patient and his care within the institution. This is particularly distressful when the net effects of such changes are relatively minimal and may already be agreed to by those at the operating levels. This problem relates to earlier comments about organizational structure and communications. Personnel must be ready and willing to make changes if programs are to develop naturally and on a timely basis. An environment should be developed in which change is expected, if not encouraged, not for change's sake, but for the opportunity it brings to improve service to patients. This requires participation by all those affected so that results are optimized and potential problems are anticipated.

Earlier I referred to specialization as an element that has added significantly to the complexity of hospital operation. The same specialization sometimes creates barriers to effective patient care. If a person who performs a test, draws blood from a patient, or cleans a patient's room does it solely because it is his job, he helps perpetuate a self-serving atmosphere. Many times an institution has tremendous personnel resources, but they are seldom coordinated to maximize patient care. The importance of each person, regardless of function, and of his attitude toward the patient must not be underestimated. It is up to all of us to express our concern for the patient in many little ways, as well as through the effective performance of our special skills. This is the basis of good patient care and the most effective way to demonstrate we are not a self-serving institution.

In evaluating self-serving tendencies of institutions, it is perhaps appropriate to also acknowledge conflicts between multiple purposes within a public service organization. The traditional functions of research, education, and patient care, as espoused by the average hospital, may raise questions regarding the optimization of patient-serving capabilities. Research interests and educational concerns ultimately must be considered on a competitive basis with patient care program needs. In these instances, however, in the appropriately motivated organization the ultimate effect on a patient care program should relate more to quantity than to quality, assuring that the care extended is as comprehensive and effective as possible. Let us, therefore, expect competition between programs within an organization, but not compromise on the essential elements of good patient care. Strong research and educational efforts ultimately contribute to improved patient care techniques.

UNDERLYING PATIENT-SERVING ELEMENT

I have cited several examples of ways in which a self-serving image can be perpetuated, restricting the effectiveness of a patient care program. I have also acknowledged that there are methods to reverse the detrimental elements, permitting the essential functioning of the organization to continue while maintaining a patient-serving environment. In each of these examples and in any potential self-serving situation, one underlying element determines whether the patient is ultimately well served. That element is individual patient concern. In each situation in which a decision is to be made, if there is concern for the effect that action has on a patient, the germ of institutional self-service cannot grow. If there is a faithful attempt to maximize the results of our labor, to communicate and participate cooperatively with all others involved in patient care, and to improve our efforts on behalf of patients, this or any other institution cannot be accused of being self-serving. It is up to us, whatever our role. It is up to you.

REFERENCES

1. Drucker, P. F.: Management: Tasks, Responsibilities, Practices. Harper & Row, New York, 1974.
2. Wren, G. R.: Modern Health Administration. University of Georgia Press, Athens, 1974.

The Conflicts Between the Personal Needs of the Staff and the Ideal of Humane Patient Treatment

CHAPTER 6

Introduction

LOIS POITRAS

The first afternoon session introduced many conflicts and ideas which served as the basis for discussions in our sessions. Most people who enter the health care services enter it to help, to cure, to provide comfort. But this cannot always be done at M. D. Anderson with the type of patients we deal with. A lot of personal problems and conflicts needed to be discussed. The first author in this section, Annabelle Chavez, is the head nurse on the pediatric floor. She was graduated from St. Joseph Hospital School of Nursing and has been associated with Anderson for some time. She has extensive experience in dealing with the cancer patient. The second author is Margaret Buchorn, who has a master's degree from The University of Chicago. She is a social psychotherapist who has been connected with the Department of Pediatrics at Anderson for many years, but who recently went into private practice for herself.

CHAPTER 7

The Concepts of Nursing in a Research Institute

ANNABELLE CHAVEZ

Those who work in a research institute need a clear understanding of all the participating departments. The goals of the Department of Nursing are three: 1) to provide safe, quality nursing care to inpatients and outpatients, 2) to provide in-service and continuing education for our nursing staff, and 3) to cooperate and participate in clinical research programs and to initiate nursing research. We nurses must recognize the impact of cancer on the patient and the family, and their physical, emotional, social, economic, and spiritual needs. We must promote and provide safe, individualized, quality nursing care for each patient.

When people learn that I work in a research institute, their reactions are varied, often negative. The words "depressing," "death," "grieving," and "sorrow" are frequently used. Many times I find myself explaining to people why I am working at M. D. Anderson. I tell them I believe that, through research, someday we will find more cures for these diseases. I deeply feel that I am an integrated part of an active, dynamic institute. Nursing in such an institute requires constant learning of new techniques, and planning and implementing nursing care. It can be a very rewarding experience. We try to offer the best nursing care that we know and provide a sound basis in learning experiences for the new nurse. Sometimes it is a hard discipline and a challenge to our emotions, because we are constantly dealing with pain, grief, death, and mutilating surgery. A nurse must learn to understand and accept her own emotions and feelings in order to help the cancer patient.

The nurse finds constant challenges in her role. What follows is an outline of some of the specific problems encountered in nursing in a research institution. Some occur in all nursing settings, but most are either accentuated in our special environment or unique to research and cancer patients.

The relationship between nurse, patient, and parent begins with the nursing assessment at admission. The admitting nurse collects and records management information for each patient. She notes the patient's habits, hobbies, favorite foods, and toys. She watches for any physical impairment in order to make adequate adjustment. We want to make the patient's stay as pleasant and painless as possible. The institution provides a full-time schoolteacher. We allow patients to wear their own clothes. Weekly parties are held with entertainment. Frequently patients are allowed home passes to break the confinement of the hospital and to keep them in contact with reality outside the hospital.

The nurse works closely with the physician, patient, family, medical-social services, chaplain, dietitian, and others in carrying out the plan for diagnosis, treatment, rehabilitation, and follow-up.

Once the diagnosis of cancer is established, a progression of problems is met by the patient, family, and medical staff. These problems include diagnosis, chronic adjustment to the disease, and often death and grieving. The nurse faces the challenges of the specialized institution. First, she has to give new, investigational drugs and observe the patient to add to the new knowledge of these treatments. These drugs have been approved by the investigational drug committee composed of doctors, nurses, and pharmacists, but they can affect the patient in many different and unexpected ways, often making him sicker, with new problems to face. The child will almost invariably require multiple venipunctures, even as the veins become more difficult to reach.

Sicker patients are more demanding. For the extremely ill, there are sophisticated machines, such as ventilators and oxygen equipment, and these require close monitoring. As the child's condition worsens, both parents and other relatives begin to stay. The room becomes congested and it is at times impossible to move around freely and provide adequate nursing care. Many times the parents do not want the nurse to perform procedures that may cause the child more discomfort. The nurse must take time to explain every action she has to take. When a child is moved to a semiprivate or private room, the other children are usually quite aware that these changes are taking place, and realize the impending death.

New problems are produced by long-term management of the chronic patient. The traditional parental role of protection is challenged and the parents feel useless, resentful, and yet want and need the competence of the staff. As the hospital stay lengthens, the parents become more apprehensive and depressed. These feelings show in their dealings with hospital personnel and other parents and are sometimes aggravated by the isolation or separation from spouses or siblings. Sometimes parents have mixed feelings in dealing with the sick child. We have a small kitchen for parents on our floor so they can cook patients' favorite foods. This kitchen is stocked and managed by the mothers. It becomes a source of many problems and an outlet for hostility when proper cleaning is not done, supplies are not accounted for, and responsibility is dodged.

The nurse must learn to deal with death and dying. She must help parents with the feelings they are experiencing. While she attempts to cope with the physical and emotional problems of the patient and the family, she continues to be responsible for the other patients on the floor. The small child will usually reflect the attitudes of the family. The teenager is more complex because he is forming his own attitudes and plans for the future. The nurse must be prepared for the times when the sequence in the stages of death and dying described by Elizabeth Kübler-Ross is not followed.[1] The mother may stop attending to the dying child and allow hospital personnel to take over, and the medical staff may not visit the dying child as much. The nurse becomes responsible for the physical and spiritual comfort of the child and family twenty-four hours a day.

New protocols are instituted constantly. Physicians' orders are complex based on these protocols. They include frequent weighings, bone marrow aspirations, administration of chemotherapeutic drugs on timed schedules, close monitoring of vital signs, and careful observation for specific side effects. Sometimes protocols are difficult to meet because of the size of the staff, the ward routine, and the physical environment. The nurse should have a definite input into the writing of protocols. She must be practical in applying and selecting a sensible plan and in using adequate equipment and personnel for the patient's welfare.

Communication between the many levels of the medical and nursing staffs remains a challenge. In our institution, shift reports between nurses are made on tape recorders and during walking rounds. Daily rounds with the medical staff help communicate the many needs of the patient. Communication between other hospital departments and the nursing staff is another constant challenge. The pediatric nurse must be practical in fitting her patient into the hurried scheduling of x-rays, radiotherapy, and so on. Fortunately, parents usually accompany children to these departments.

The physical ward is a constraint. There are four beds in each ward room and two ward rooms share a bathroom. Storage room for suitcases and personal articles is limited. With one parent (and sometimes two) staying with each child, the ward rooms become quite crowded. One conference room is next to the nurses' station. This is used for nurses' shift reports, doctors' conferences, in-service training lectures, and conferences with parents. More conference rooms are needed to meet the needs of our Social Service Department, nursing reporting, and conferences. We desperately need a special room for consoling bereaved families.

Our Nursing Department feels constant pressure from other departments as well as from some hospital policies. Rules forbidding food service to families in the hospital rooms and setting strict visiting hours may cause hardships. We are aware of this and realize this is what makes us different from the general hospital.

Our nursing goals and plans for the care of each patient are developed and based on research projects and the needs of the individual patient. Nurses should take the initiative and seek information from the medical staff and from our research library. We should attempt to attend all staff meetings and workshops to improve our knowledge so that we can give better service to our patients. We should also try to learn to appreciate the human aspects of each individual patient and family in a spiritual way. In this way we can offer the comfort they need.

Finally, we have to continually help new nurses, physicians, and other staff members to answer the questions: "Why is all this necessary? What is the rationale behind these many protocols? Why prolong the life of this hopelessly ill patient?" I feel that a human life is very precious and we can offer hope to these patients. If we can ease pain and offer periods of remission, some of our goals will have been met.

REFERENCE

1. Kübler-Ross, E.: On Death and Dying. Macmillan, New York, 1969.

CHAPTER 8

The Patient's Needs: A Twenty-four-hour Demand in an Eight-hour Day

MARGARET BUCHORN

The topic of this chapter, the patient's needs, could be approached in several different ways. The term "patient" in the context of this presentation means the hospitalized child and the caregivers who are hospitalized with him. These caregivers (whom I shall call parents, although other adults are included) are in effect hospitalized. In truth, the child who is physically ill may suffer less than the well parent from the confinement. We are all aware that when we feel sick enough, interest in our surroundings and other happenings is minimal. It is well known that the progress of a convalescence is measured by the patient's complaints about heretofore tolerated procedures and urgent desire to return to normal activities; thus we measure both physical and emotional health. How much more, then, does the physically sound parent experience the confinement, the removal from normal routine and interests, brought about by residing with his child on a cancer ward?

Parents sometimes compare their residency on 6-West to confinement in a mental hospital or a jail. Neither of these analogies is precise, although there are similarities. Most persons confined to mental hospitals are there because they themselves or someone close to them considered them overwhelmed by the stresses of everyday living. Many such patients find sanctuary and comfort in their confinement. Those persons imprisoned by the state for crimes are compelled to remain incarcerated for a designated length of time and can usually adjust accordingly. The 6-West parents, far from being overwhelmed by reality, are usually very much involved with it, aware of the many urgent outside demands which need their attention, and impatient to be free again to deal with these. The continuing uncertainty of the duration of their stay is another especially aggravating factor, as it makes planning impossible. Parents are not required to reside on 6-West by any necessity other than their own love for the child and sense of responsibility.

Our present inclination to view the body as the entire person, rather than as only one aspect of a person, leads us to many erroneous assumptions. When a person's body develops problems, when it houses an illness or functions improperly, that person correctly takes it to a physician, whose particular expertise is repairing or improving body function. But both parties—the patient and the physician—have come to attribute many other functions unrelated to this area of expertise to the physician. Historically this has grown out of the human need for certainty, a need which formerly found assurance in the supernatural powers attributed to the witch doctor and the authority invested in the priest.

The whole issue of whether it is morally and philosophically sound for an entire family to give over control and direction of all of their lives to an institution because of the physical illness of one family member is an issue I can only raise. I have never been able to resolve it satisfactorily for myself. I have behaved as if this presumption were valid out of my indisputable knowledge that, if my own child were an inmate of 6-West, with a body invaded by cancer, I could only remain with my child. So I proceed as if this presumption that patients' families should be under our care and thus at our disposal is valid. To enumerate the many burdens and crises of these families would surely be superfluous. Everyone is intimately and painfully familiar with the many special demands and strains on such families—emotional, social, and financial. Each of us has grieved for some family special to us or been inspired by the heroism rising out of tragedy. Therefore, I choose to approach my task of illuminating patients' needs by exploring ways that this painful living situation can be made meaningful and enriching.

To quote Pogo Possum in the memorable cartoon strip: "We have met the enemy and he is us." It is always so much easier to discuss a patient's needs than to look to our own needs and resources. It would be presumptuous in the extreme for anyone to propose that a hospital unit could attempt to meet all needs of all patients. Not only presumptuous but absurd. Yet I fear that at times we proceed as if that were a reasonable goal. Confinement to 6-West will not cause inadequate, limited personalities to become strong and free, nor will it bring about happy marriages or achieving students, if the capacities are not brought to us. A reasonable goal, rather, is to take this confinement, which is basically hard, bitter, and destructive to human development, and attempt to foster a positive, growth-producing, and life-affirming experience—in short, a therapeutic community. This is no small task; indeed, it may well be an impossible one. For any hope of success, the joint energies and efforts of each of us must be enlisted. As I understand, that is precisely the reason the Pediatric Workshop was organized. My definition of a therapeutic community is a controlled environmental situation in which people interact for their mutual therapeutic benefit, and in which observations and interventions of all staff members are important to the therapeutic process.

The concept of a therapeutic community grew up in the 1950's in mental hospitals. The ideal is that the patient is surrounded by a community of loving, well intentioned staff members, each contributing the best of his own skills and competence. Often this ideal degenerates into a sterile, competitive arena filled with individuals vying for authority and the patient's first allegiance. In the typical conforming climate of the 1950's the ideal was replaced by the concept of a group of variously trained and equipped individuals who were interchangable in their functioning.

Can a therapeutic community ever be achieved in a society in which competitive, materialistic achievement is extolled as the greatest glory? The so-called counterculture of the 1960's, with its emphasis on loving relationships and experiments in communal living, offered some hope. Certainly if the family unit as we know it is to survive, it requires bolstering by society as a substitute for the clan or extended family. Is it possible for the community to sustain or bolster without demanding control and regulation, which have always characterized assistance throughout history, however benevolent in intent? Is it possible for a cancer center to offer a supportive, helpful milieu to patients without demanding submission to its requirements and management?

We begin with the recognition that most of us work not out of a feeling of commitment and joy, but rather out of a desperation, a need to feed and sustain our bodies, a feeling often of being victims without choice. By the time we reach the age of employment, most of us have been so programmed by our culture that it takes much time, effort, and luck for us to perceive who we really are, as opposed to how we are supposed to be. The dim realization that we are not authentic, true to our own being, forces us to attempt to feed on others and assuage our own anxiety at feeling so miserable by belittling or destroying our fellow human beings.

How many times has each of us observed the competitive vying on 6-West, each representative of a different discipline in hot pursuit of the closest relationship with the patient, a nugget of "secret information," a particular claim to intimacy? Yet each of us expresses his own being in different ways to different persons in different situations. We reveal different aspects of ourselves to a loved one, a child, or a policeman—at least I hope each of us does. Why is it so difficult for us to acknowledge this aspect of human nature in patients? The same mother who confides her panic in the middle of the night may well express optimistic assurance the following sunny morning. This is neither contradictory nor hypocritical—nor necessarily revealing of any special relationships with the recipient of her verbalizations.

Then there is what I call the "noble savage" concept, which implies that the less sophisticated the staff member, the more helpful he is to the patient. Inherent in this idea is the constantly disproved but constantly advanced notion that the quantity of a relationship in some way substitutes for quality. This notion is most widely applied to the mother—child relationship, in which constant physical presence is often extolled as the essential ingredient. Surely each of us is aware that we are often physically present with others without being present in any other sense. So the "noble savage" school promotes the idea that the staff member who is physically with the patient the greatest amount of time has the closest relationship with him. In most hospital situations this would be the aide. Now it is often true that the aide is the recipient of many confidences the patient has not shared with other staff members. In addition to availability, many aides are warm, understanding individuals, but I venture there are other factors.

Those of us who have been consultants to elementary schools have frequently heard that the janitor is the person most confided in by the children. Aside from the sympathetic attitudes of the individual aide or janitor, which can not be overlooked, I submit that at least part of the explanation of this is that these are persons able to let the patient or the child be. The aide or janitor is usually perceived not only as a person available and comfortable, but as someone relatively powerless in that particular hierarchy, and therefore "safe." The child, for example, is secure that the janitor will not feel compelled to call in his parents for a school conference and make a "big deal" out of betraying his confidences.

When staff members see themselves in competitive roles, struggling to control the patient or his situation, they often view other staff members as intrusive busybodies. A sad example perhaps can help clarify this. An infuriated, despairing chaplain confided to me that he had been enlisted by the adult children of a comatose old man to intercede with their father's physician. The family felt very frustrated by their inability to communicate to the physician their wish to discontinue the mechanical life-support measures. The chaplain's appropriate, courteous presentation of this viewpoint was met by the physician with enraged accusations that the children were only concerned with their financial benefit, that the chaplain was meddling in a situation in which he did not rightfully belong, and that he, the physician (by sustaining this comatose sub-life), was the only friend and advocate the old man had. This physician's possessiveness and grandiosity was only an extreme expression of an all-too-common attitude. The only possible answer to the question, "Who does the patient belong to?" is, "To *no one.*" Each of us belongs only to himself and when we cannot act in our own behalf, our relatives are socially and legally sanctioned actors for us.

This particular family had felt the need of enlisting one authority figure (minister) to prevail for them against another authority figure (physician). No one can deny that the physician has been the supreme authority figure in this country for the past seventy-odd years. This is rapidly changing, even in Texas. We can hope that a golden mean of mutual respect and honest dealing between patient and physician will evolve. The physician earned his position as an authority figure in the hospital and in our society by a commendable willingness to assume responsibility and leadership. This entailed long, grueling hours as well as life-and-death decisions. The complexity of our present way of living makes it impossible for any one group of experts to hold a patent on knowledge. This seems self-evident, yet we all know it is very difficult for an entrenched group to alter characteristic ways of operating, and perhaps it is naive to anticipate that such a group would voluntarily relinquish power or status. Yet if our ideal of a therapeutic community is to be approached, such a relinquishment is necessary.

Perhaps a further illustration will help clarify my position. At one of the meetings with parents on 6-West, a mother began discussing her concern about a school-related problem of a well child at home. The young pediatrician conducting the meeting with me referred her to her local pediatrician when she was able to return home again. I disagreed. It seemed obvious to me that the place to begin exploring a school-related problem was the school. Then one might appropriately proceed to any number of specialists for attention, a speech therapist, a Boy Scout leader, or a psychotherapist. To assume that this mother needed the permission or guidance of a physician in this situation was as inappropriate, in my mind, as to ask a physician to refer her to a tax lawyer or a dance instructor.

This persistent belief in ownership of the patient is one of the greatest obstacles to the development of a therapeutic community. The inability of the physician to share responsibility and to acknowledge the contributions of other disciplines is a real impediment. The traditional hospital structure, in which the physician snaps out orders and the nurses and others unquestioningly carry them out, is the antithesis of a therapeutic community in which mutual respect and real coopera- tion are the truly essential ingredients. This fact was brought sharply into focus on 6-West with the initiation of a weekly meeting for personnel, the expressed purpose of which was sharing information and discussing problem situations. This opportunity to work together was embraced enthusiastically by all staff members except some of the physicians. Some interns and residents participated freely and produc- tively, but others showed by their absence or attitudes how threatening such a change in role status was to them.

Even cursory observation will reveal that most institutions are run to meet the needs of the staff rather than the patients. When one considers the physicial surroundings at Anderson, it is difficult to imagine that anyone's needs are being met—except possibly those of the Legislative Budget Committee. A work situation in which no one has space or privacy can only be detrimental to the interests of all. Neces- sary routines can preclude a meeting place for a family whose child has just died or for a discussion by an important consultant for which a group of interested specialists have left urgent concerns of their own. I hope many of the constant, daily irritations taken out on each other or patients will be eliminated by more spacious quarters.

But removal of the cause of a bad habit does not always remove the habit. Some of our destructive ways of functioning together can, we hope, be left behind. One that I feel is never justified is discussing a patient's situation within earshot of other patients or casual passersby. This practice coexists with the obsessive concern that the patient might read his own medical chart, which presumably is entirely about him and in which his interest should be paramount. Although patients may know much more about each other's personal situations than the staff ever learns, it remains inexcusable for them to glean such information from the staff by overhearing it or by gossip. My personal creed is that any patient is entitled to all information about himself and none concerning another patient. If I hold views about a patient that I consider would be damaging for him to learn, I had best look to my relationship with him, rather than assume that in my omnipotence I can judge what is best for another human being.

While the professional staff are somewhat aware of these physical handicaps to their own functioning, they often are strangely insensitive to the implications to the patients. Such seemingly small, yet important, niceties as knocking on doors before entering or speaking before pulling back drawn curtains, which would demonstrate a respect for human dignity, are ignored. I doubt if many of us would barge into another's home, least of all a bedroom, without prior announcement. To the patient living there, the hospital room is his home. My only explanation to indignant parents regarding this rudeness is that the hospital personnel perceive the room as their office or domain, in which the patient is the intruder. Another constant source of resentment to patients is the gratuitous opinion expressed by staff members about personal habits or preferences. Such matters as hair length, dress, or food preferences are criticized as if there were a right or wrong in personal taste. This smugness is most easily spotted when we deal with patients from other cultures or races. It is perhaps more difficult to discern with patients more like ourselves of whom we subtly disapprove.

A vexing obstacle in trying to establish a supportive milieu is the wide disagreement among staff members as to what represents appropriate behavior and what should be the staff posture toward generally unacceptable behavior. I see no advantage, in our attempts to be accepting of other human beings, to characterize them as "psychotic" rather than "no-good." Both labels express our own distaste for the individual designated and our inability to be at ease with him.

The best illustration I know involves the basic issue of an adult remaining with a hospitalized child. The official policy of the institution, eloquently and sincerely voiced by the head of the Department of Pediatrics, is that one adult may stay with each child at all times, but there is no requirement for any adult to ever stay. If the care-givers elect to visit the child at certain hours, the Department of Pediatrics assumes full responsibility for the child's medical care and general well-being, just as if the institution limited visiting to two hours on Sunday afternoon (which only a few years ago was the officially approved quota). Most parents elect to stay with their hospitalized child, but woe unto the parent who does not. Such a parent is met with tremendous group disapproval from staff and other parents, often just at a time when that parent is most in need of understanding or at least consideration. Unanimity of opinion about life-styles and preferences is never possible, nor would it be desirable. But fundamental respect for the right of another human being to choose his own way—even an erroneous way by our lights—appears to me to be essential.

Another common example is the "double message" transmitted when we give intellectual lip service to principles we have not integrated emotionally. An example: Most people working on 6-West really believe that a mother who has been confined with a cranky, whiney, ill child for weeks or months needs some relief. The Volunteer Department goes to great lengths to facilitate this. When the weary parent finally goes out for an evening, she often returns to a barrage of criticism from other parents and staff if the child has cried or become ill. This, to a parent already feeling torn about confinement and guilty at leaving the child, can be devastating. The expressed hostility increases geometrically if the brief time outside is suspected of including indulgence in alcohol or sex. Realistically a momentary indulgence in either of these activities may well increase the parent's capacity to be a "good parent."

One of the misunderstandings expressed in a planning session for the Pediatric Workshop was that it was to be a "love-in" or "encounter sessions." Such was not our charge, although personally I hope both more love and more encountering have come out of the weekend. My more modest ambition is that each of us may be more inclined to examine his own head, to determine which needs are appropriately gratified through our interrelations with other staff or with patients and which are not.

SECTION IV

The Truly Cured Child

CHAPTER 9

Introduction

CHARLES SHAW

I was a little bit curious as to whether Dr. van Eys had any specific intent in assigning me the section on the truly cured child. I suspect he did. I am sure he is well aware that in many schools of psychotherapy the concept of cure, of being sick or of being well, is rejected. The point is that this medical model, sick versus well, implies a discontinuous state, while the field of psychiatry sees mental health as a continuum from degrees of adjustment to degrees of maladjustment. This has been well delineated by Thomas Szasz in his book, *The Myth of Mental Illness.*[1] On the other hand, with a physical disease such as cancer we know there is a discontinuum: a person either has cancer or he doesn't. Sometimes he may not know it, sometimes determination of this is difficult, but there is a state of well-being, of being cured of cancer. I do not belong to any single school of psychiatry; I do not even belong to psychiatry any more. But I am comfortable with the concept of sickness versus health in the field of mental disease as well as physical disease, and I certainly feel we see people who are clearly mentally ill. I have even been willing to write on some charts that, in my opinion, this person is mentally normal, mentally well.

We talked in this last session of the conference about the child and whether or not he is cured. I did not know what Dr. van Eys was going to say, but I expected he would ask us to think about both the physical and emotional aspects. I think it was fitting that, after Dr. van Eys' presentation, we heard from parents of the children. We need them.

REFERENCE

1. Szasz, T. S.: The Myth of Mental Illness: Foundations of a Theory of Personal Conduct. Rev. ed., Harper & Row, New York, 1974.

CHAPTER 10

What Do We Mean by "The Truly Cured Child"?

JAN VAN EYS

Curing cancer is the goal that we set for ourselves. While it is clear that "cancer" is a term for a group of diseases, one common denominator is that all patients with cancer have cells growing out of control by the rest of their bodies, and that such growth can be destructive to the point of death. In that light, cure of cancer means either eradication of the malignant cells or at least bringing these cells under control again.

It was not very long ago that cancer in children was an acutely fatal illness. Medical care was aimed at ameliorating the consequences of the disease, with only occasional attempts at cure. A few decades ago modern technology, biochemistry, and surgery made a multimodal attack on childhood cancer possible, so that we now talk about cures as a norm.[1]

This spectacular success was achieved rapidly and yet painstakingly. Rapidly, in hindsight: chemotherapy began in the 1940's. Painstakingly, because the trial-and-error method of adapting theoretical ideas to practical patient care failed to save many children who were diagnosed at times when most attempts at cure were unsuccessful. Even now only a few cancers are routinely curable. Pediatricians can always proudly point to Wilms' tumor. Yet to date we have to admit our poor results with brain tumors.

Nevertheless, remarkable and gratifying progress came about through clinical research, by trial and error.* Such clinical research was not hard-hearted, but the best we had to offer to the children: namely, a genuine concern about the problem. But to avoid excessive errors, sights had to be set in a limited way. First of all, results of therapy had to be measured against length of survival. When prolongation of survival became the norm, a more refined criterion had to be found. Disease-free survival or length of initial remission became the measures of therapeutic effectiveness. That concession to success was the first acknowledgment of the quality of survival. In fact, such success became the expected, so that mere survival became decried as unworthy of the human patient. As life became prolonged, evaluation of the impact of disease on mental health came into focus. Children lived longer, and often surprisingly disease free, but they still died. Therefore attention was directed to the dying patient. This was a significant development

---

*It may seem callous to describe the seeking for cure as a trial-and-error method, but a recent article by Thomas defines the method as the highest quality of human accomplishment.[2]

which recognized that the efforts expended on the patient should not cease when biological failure occurs. A recent workshop at the Institute of Religion in Houston called this new attitude "Responsible Steward-ship of Human Life."[3]

But medicine progressed. Continuous complete remissions became indefinite in length. Therapy began to be discontinued, and continuous, complete, unmaintained remissions are now not infrequent. It may be too early to call these children "cured" because the certainty of cure will not come for many decades. But the concept of a period of risk defines a span of time within which most, if not all, recurrences occur. If that concept remains valid, we have achieved in pediatric oncology a respectable number of biological cures. We have eradicated the malig-nant cells from the body of the patient.

Do we thereby have a "cured" child? In one sense, of course, we do. But do we have a truly cured child, a child who is mentally healthy and who can function at an age-appropriate level in society? Pediatrics has a unique problem. Such a cure cannot be achieved through rehabilitation, because few skills have been learned as yet. Certainly we can retrain in physical dexterity, such as relearning to walk after an amputation. However, for a child to be cured, he has to view the world with anticipation and with an eagerness to learn what his peers are learning. If that is our end point, have we indeed already achieved cures? Clearly we have not. In fact, when we focus on mental health at all we are more apt to still deal with death and dying. It is the purpose of this chapter to explore the areas in which we are failing to optimize our curative intent. It will be my thesis that this effort is a problem for all the individuals concerned with the treatment of the child: physicians, nurses, paramedical personnel, supportive volunteers, parents, and so-ciety at large.

IS A TRULY CURED CHILD
A LEGITIMATE CONCERN OF MEDICINE?

We must first examine whether we are discussing a legitimate question. A basic premise of surgery is that, given half the chance, wounds will heal. While wounds can be made to heal with minimal scars through careful attention, the wise surgeon achieves this through minimal han-dling. It could be argued that we should make an analogy. A child will develop normally, given half a chance. Therefore oncology need concern itself only with the cancer.

A recent article addressed itself indirectly to this question.[4] Black argues that a physician should not be concerned with a nebulous concept of health. Indeed, health is a concept that defines a state of complete physical, mental, and social well-being and not merely the absence of disease or infirmity. A truly cured child is a healthy child, not just a child from whom a cancer has been removed. There is a great difficulty in defining health when approaching it from the standpoint of nonhealth. However, with a specific illness there is very little problem in defining nonhealth.

Health to a particular individual is often more dependent on mental and social well-being than on arbitrary standards of physical well-being.[5] The task of medicine is first to restore optimal physical well-being, and then to allow mental and social well-being to develop. It is the task of the physician to allow that to happen, even if he cannot himself define what health is for a given patient. Black is correct that health can be beyond the scope of a given physician, but a truly cured child must be a healthy one nevertheless. A truly cured child is a legitimate end point.

The question therefore revolves around the means by which a child achieves mental and social well-being. A child's development continues when he has cancer. It may be even faster than normal under the stress of the disease. But the environment must be conducive to *normal* development. That environment is not just the one created by the parents at home but the sum total of all experiences that the child has during his illness. The child must be allowed normal development during abnormal circumstances.

Normal development requires, first, sensorimotor equipment that is as normal as possible. A blind or deaf child is handicapped in achieving normal development. It remains achievable, to be sure, but it requires considerably more effort. Second, normal development requires an environment that allows step-by-step progression. A child must select from the environment those concepts required for development from the stimuli offered. Finally, normal development requires a self-image that allows positive social interaction.

Modern medicine must attempt biological cure. But once cure is possible, its cost must be minimized to allow a healthy child. That remains a challenge to health care delivery. Therefore, we are dealing with not only a legitimate question but even a necessary one.

IS THE HEALTHY CHILD
ACHIEVABLE UNDER CURRENT MANAGEMENT?

There was little difficulty in changing from increased survival time, to prolonged remission time, and then to indefinite remission time as a goal of therapy. Why, then, should we now have a problem in achieving the ultimate goal, a truly cured child? The pervading attitude is preoccupation with the quality of life. Because we frequently feel that the quality of life may be inferior, we as cancer caregivers are more often perturbed by last-ditch efforts than we are by peaceful death. We often prepare parents and patients for the demise. It is, after all, easier to tolerate dying as the norm and reap the occasional cure as reward rather than expect cure and accept death as failure.

We have thereby done two things. First, we have allowed ourselves the luxury of euthanasia. We decry physical euthanasia, but psychological euthanasia is no better. Telling a patient prematurely that he is going to die becomes a self-fulfilling prophesy. That does not mean that telling the truth is not desirable, but the truth must be objective, and the motives behind rushing the death prediction are often far removed from those engendered by objectivity.

Second, we have now a new iatrogenic disease, what Easson called the "Lazarus syndrome."[6,7] A family is emotionally prepared for the loss of a child, yet the child returns to generate an unmanagable upheaval of feelings and resentments. We do not usually have such extreme cases, but neither are we as yet prepared for success. We must expect our children to be cured so we can prepare ourselves to allow them to become healthy again. In so doing we are going to be hurt, because many of our children will not be cured. But we must take that next step now, because if we do not *none* of our children will be truly cured.

No matter how we eventually manage the disease called cancer, some intervention will be necessary. Even if the child is cured, his self-concept has to be put at ease with having had cancer. The cost of cure should not interfere with development. The physical cost is the problem of the child: a decreased ability to absorb out of the environment the information and stimuli to grow. But the mental cost is the problem of the caregivers, parents as well as health care deliverers. Our attitudes define to a large degree the growth in mental health of the child.

THE PHYSICAL COST OF CURE

There is no doubt that the severity of intervention can result in an equally severe physical handicap. Acute iatrogenic disease is only too well known. Marrow depression and immune suppression are always a danger of radiation and chemotherapy. There may be more delayed, organ-specific side effects: we are all familiar with pancreatitis accompanying L-asparaginase therapy, cystitis of Cytoxan, and pulmonary fibrosis of busulfan, to name but a few. If we add to these the real handicap of mutilative surgery, then it is easily seen that there are very many physical consequences of curative attempts. Since we have conceded that health does not necessarily require perfect bodily function, that mental and social well-being are more important, such gross physical consequences are only important in two ways within the context of our present discussion. First, they may threaten to undo the physical cure by resulting in iatrogenic death. Second, they may severely threaten the child's self-image.

Physical side effects are not automatically threatening to cognitive development. Rarely are the senses sufficiently impaired to hinder development. But there are exceptions. First, there are increasing reports that intensive central nervous system therapy may result in disseminating necrotizing leukoencephalopathy.[8, 9] This raises the fear that there might be subtle damage in many children. However, one study found no such long-term neuropsychological effects.[10] The issue is not clearly resolved as yet, and many more studies need to be done.

Another problem is coming to the fore. Children who are cured of one cancer are more prone to develop a second.[11] Whether this is a consequence of therapy or an expression of the inherent cancer proneness of the child is unclear, and is not an important distinction to the child. The danger of second malignancies may significantly detract from a sense of physical cure.

It is clear, therefore, that biological cures, physical eradications of disease, by present management are not often fully realized. In this sense a truly cured child may not be attainable as yet. But the impact is relatively minor compared to the other obstacles to the truly cured child generated by the mental cost of cure.

THE MENTAL COST OF THERAPY

The mental cost of therapy is severe. In discussing it we need to be careful to avoid circular reasoning. After all, health was defined as a state free of damage to social and mental performances. If therapy exacts a mental cost, we could say that a truly cured child is impossible by definition. But the cost of an item only describes payment, not necessarily attainability. Only when cost exceeds ability or willingness to pay are cost and outcome automatically linked.

The mental cost exacted is the same as the strain any chronic illness places on a child's development. The special areas in which cancer may be unique have been recently reviewed.[11, 12]   Briefly, one can discern areas of conflict in delayed development, vocational alterations, poor self-image, and adjustment problems in parents and siblings. Almost all these costs are exacted by the caring adults, who have a great problem seeing the child as he is. We adults usually want the child to behave as if there were no cancer. We often hope that cure will remove a cancer so that the child will be brought back as if nothing had happened. Conversely, we sometimes treat the child as if the cancer were all. We treat the child as the poor suffering one, not allowing him to be himself, as normal as any other child in spirit. Both of our attitudes create despair in the child. It is one of the most obvious examples of the forms of despair that Kierkegaard describes in his book, *The Sickness unto Death*: despair is being what you do not want to be, or not being what you want to be.[13] To take the cancer away from the child is to deny that child a major aspect of his reality. To focus on the cancer only is to deny the child the normal world.

This treatment is no different from that which any handicapped child suffers from adults. Cancer is almost always now a chronic disease, no matter what the outcome. There is, consequently, a great similarity between the problems of the cancer-stricken child and those of the handicapped child. The limited ability of family, siblings and parents alike, to cope with the additional stress may even require psychiatric intervention.[14] Not all the problems are caused by the family. The child with a chronic illness may have visual-motor problems that stem from the illness rather than a specific handicap.[15] Yet within all the framework of the chronic illness and the coping behavior that is required from the whole family, it must be stressed that the demands on the health care professionals are no different. The difficulty in being involved with a child for whom one wishes a better fate results in frequent assumptions of reactions by the child that reflect not the personality of the child but the fears of the adult.[16]

It was suggested that the child will develop, given half a chance. If the analogy with wound healing is valid, then difficulties may more often be created by excessive interference than by allowing the child to take his own development in hand. However, a child can learn from the environment only by choosing from what is available. If the environment allows no healthy choice, development will be warped, no matter what the child's potential. Therefore, allowing a child to develop on his own emphatically does not mean that there are never circumstances in which intervention is desirable. There may be pathological adjustments in family and patient alike. In some infrequent cases the child has disease- or treatment-induced handicaps in cognitive skills, so that he is unable to maximally benefit from the environment. More frequently one observes the agony of adults watching a child struggle with a task that he has to master but that they could do easier and faster. Many handle that situation well, but overprotection of the handicapped child is a very frequent problem. As a result, the child is not allowed to learn a difficult skill.

In the same way the child with cancer has to learn to be himself with cancer, and we should not take his world in our hands to make it easier for him. Even if we could ease his burden in the short term, this clearly is counterproductive in the long run. Yet we so often add to the cost of cancer by making the child act in ways less painful to us. The best example comes from the current interest in death and dying. Kübler-Ross has described a number of stages that are recognizable in the dying patient. Now, however, patients are expected to follow that path because the predictability is mentally easier to bear for the caregivers. Some recent voices have pointed out the self-serving attitude inherent in such a view.[18] In the case of the chronically ill patient, similar dynamics are at work in the stressed family. Many problems are raised for the caring adult in accepting the chronically ill child. If that child is in danger of death the problems are compounded. The adult often feels guilt in being unable to protect the child from such devastating disease and its consequences.

It is precisely here that the interaction between child and adult sets in motion a dynamic cause and effect. We adults perceive a poor quality of life and try to make amends to the child in any way that will make us feel better. For instance, a parent refuses to discipline because the expected reaction would result in the parent feeling guilty of coercing the child toward something thought to be unpleasant. This is only a minor example, and only used to bring the point home because it is the most obvious one.

But the burden does not lie primarily on the parents. It is, of course, true that the sick child must be treated in such a way that the whole family is alleviated to the greatest extent possible from the burden the chronic illness imposes. But this results in a very large variety of care postures, since the needs of families are as many as there are people. Rather, the burden lies to a great degree on the medical care system, because we act in stereotyped manners and lack adaptability. We are just as threatened by our feelings as the parents are. Our interventions are often equally self-serving in that they are designed to minimize our feelings of inadequacy.

There are many books that give advice on the care of children in hospitals. The classical guidelines are given by the American Academy of Pediatrics.[19] However, that information is geared toward the incidentally sick child. The chronically ill child, especially one with a life-threatening illness, poses problems far beyond the usual needs because he enters a new reality when the diagnosis of cancer is given. When a child has an uncomplicated appendectomy, the illness can be treated as a transient event. Such an event will always be remembered, to be sure, but the child can be master and incorporate it without upheaval of his whole life, life expectancy, or goal orientation. But again, it is not primarily the perception of the child that matters. The younger child especially sees little difference between the small illness and the life-threatening or chronic one.[20] The problem lies in the attitude of the caring adults, who see that difference very clearly and react quite differently toward the different children.

The mental cost of therapy is therefore very real, but it is in no small measure exacted from the child by the adult. A child with cancer is treated as an exceptional child, even though he wants desperately to be normal.

THE CAUSES OF THE PROBLEM

A severe accusation has thus been leveled at the health care delivery system in pediatric oncology. It may be thought that it applies only to cancer care, but that is not so. It can apply to the care for any illness in which the cure rate is finite but not consistent, and in which the cure is achieved through long and painstaking treatment. However, if these were the only underlying causes for the accusation, one could argue that the problem will be self-solving. As soon as cure becomes ever more routine, the truly cured child will automatically emerge. It is not that simple, however, because the cure has to be recognized. Today's pioneers become the conservatives of tomorrow. The early comprehensive cancer centers were indeed pioneers. They diligently strove to bring about their own demise. But very soon they became self-serving: research became the end rather than the means by which the goal was reached. This problem is not peculiar to the cancer center but is a general phenomenon in human endeavors.

The patient care aspects of a cancer center are no different. The challenges of nursing the patient who might die are so great that it is hard to nurse a patient who might live. The emotional and physical investment in the care of the patient is so great that the caregiver has to protect himself. We all have to have a means by which we can cope with what we are doing. Our work includes the dying patient, the patient who is mutilated, and even the patient who is truly cured after long and arduous effort. All of us have to come to grips with that through the formulation of a belief structure, a *Weltanschauung*, that makes it possible to cope with the unanswerable. After all, the care that we are asked to give is overwhelming. It is possible to remain aloof, to just do a task rather than give health care. But it is impossible to befriend a child and not immediately be faced with all the questions about human existence that religion and philosophy have struggled with since time immemorial.

Most of us do become involved with at least one child. To make our belief system work, we then must pretend to ourselves that the child is totally ours, that whatever happens to that child conforms to whatever is best for him in our eyes. Of course we know that that cannot be and we rationalize most of the time the diversity of interpretation of the unknowable: we admit that the various beliefs are equally valid. But we all come up again to that one special child who deserves so much better than we can apparently give, and the best that we can give is our belief in what is right, just, and ethical.

The consequence is that we all begin to believe we are the primary contact for that child. This belief is strengthened by the fact that children do select a friend in times of need. When a child is dying, and the world becomes too fast for him to cope, he will usually select one or at most a very few adults as friends and confidantes. But he selects a friend, a fellow human being, not a nurse or a doctor. That is over-powering. A friendship is a gift and a burden. It is much easier to translate the friendship into a professional demand.

A great struggle begins as a consequence. Each profession feels primarily responsible for the child and it becomes very difficult to generate a team. In a sense, our success has become our downfall. When cancer care was an all-or-none affair, it was easy. A child was cured or he died. Now a child lives five years, and he is cured or he dies. To become involved with that child as a team is very hard. Yet a team does not preclude friendship, quite the contrary. There are so many patients, and so few of us, that every team member is necessary to develop friendships. But in the past that was thought unprofessional—you had to remain first and foremost a doctor or a nurse.

To reconcile these two demands, all professions have considered themselves the primary generators of health in the child. The doctor considers the biological cure so paramount that he often ignores or, worse, degrades everything else. The nurse thinks that she could be considered the pivot because she is frequently the instrument through which curative agents are administered, and at the same time she is the primary support of the child. The social and mental health services consider the child in society so important, compared to the hospital setting, that they see health care delivery as a minor part of the child's needs. The pastoral services think that the spirit is paramount, so they become the purveyors of health. Yet the diverse needs of the patient make everyone eventually fall back on the common denominator, the presumed psychological needs of all patients, rather than the special needs of a special child or family. As a result, the duplication of presumed roles becomes competitive. In addition, all feel threatened when called upon to restructure their roles within the bounds of their specific reasons for participating in the care of the child in the first place.*

All this may sound like unfounded exaggeration, yet examples abound. For instance, the pastoral counseling service concentrates frequently on the general mental health of the patient rather than on displaying its special calling. There are exceptions, but this is generally true for the Protestant denominations. Another example is the nursing services. As often as not the nursing training courses deal with psychological assessment of the patient rather than with specific nursing skills that might be needed.

Examples do not prove an assertion, but the assertion is not provable in the scientific sense of the word. Rather, it is a hypothesis that can be tested if we want to make the consequent predictions and compare them with the experience of reality.

STEPS TOWARD THE TRULY CURED CHILD

So far we have said that the truly cured child is a healthy one, with social, mental, and physical well-being. We have also said that the child needs to achieve this through normal development, and that one of the greatest handicaps toward normal development is the adult's concept of his illness, resulting in a self-concept and environment that are counterproductive. Finally it was argued that the health care delivery team's misconception of his illness came about through the blurring of the line between professional role and personal involvement.

The prediction, then, is that a change in our attitude toward the professional role might break the current impasse. There is a model, namely, psychiatric treatment units. In such units the aim is the development of a mentally healthy child. There are differences, of course. The mentally ill child is sick and has to be restored to health. In the child with cancer only the body is sick, and whatever mental illnes comes about is of our creation. However, the similarities are great. A mental health treatment unit is primarily concerned with bringing reality into focus. In a family setting the love of the parents and their

---

*This argument is not negated by the frequent unquestioning attitude of following the physician's guidance in medical care. While in fact the questioning is insufficient, the execution of medical orders reflects the biological aspects of care and neither detracts from nor serves as a guide to personal involvement.

authority are both accepted and not usually confused by the child if the parents show no confusion. In a mental health treatment center the roles of the various counselors are clearly delineated. Their involvement with the patient is spelled out, and patient confusion about separation and limit setting is dealt with in great detail. The problems for the caregivers are also dealt with in great depth so that they can cope with their feelings in ways that do not interfere with the task at hand: the generation of an independent human being. Some claim that a clearly delineated environment with full acceptance of the child as a person in his own right can rehabilitate even the autistic child.[21] The secret of that success lies in the attitudes of the caregivers, not in their intervention with the child. A child will indeed develop in ways that the environment allows.

The physically sick child is no different. Diffusing the role of the medical personnel is at best confusing, and at worst degrading. After all, a nurse is a nurse and a doctor a doctor. Both do things to and for the child that are good and pleasant one time and painful and frightening another time. But that has nothing to do with the love they feel toward the child. No apology is necessary for our medical care if we really believe it is the best we can devise for that child. The child is not an individual with a malignant disease totally foreign to his being, but rather a person with cancer who could not be any other person. No apology for a marrow aspiration is necessary for a leukemic child—it is part of his life because he has cancer. The procedure is performed because the physician thinks it is essential for his well-being.

The most normalizing influence in a child's life remains the consistent family. The participation of the family in the child's care demands attention to the well-being of the family as well. But most importantly, the medical team taking care of the child becomes absorbed in the child's extended family, the conceptual group of caring and nurturing adults. This is true even if the medical team is not aware of the demands placed on it by the children.

Therefore, the optimal way in which truly cured children can be achieved is through the generation of a therapeutic community. A therapeutic community implies an atmosphere and an organizational structure in which all who come into contact with the patient are part of a healing and supporting group, each with his own expertise, but acting in concerted decision making. Only in such a way can we hope to achieve the same check-and-balance system that operates in a healthy family, in which the father figure has to cease being pompous when the equal-partner mother calls him down.

In a therapeutic community there must be mutual support and role divisions. This implies the need for generating respect and a sense of equality among all professional and paraprofessional personnel, with a feeling of satisfaction on the part of all within their specific, defined roles. Such a community is achievable. It requires, however, a basic concept change in the current hierarchical structures, especially in the roles of nurses and physicians. On the one hand, the nurse needs to participate actively in decision making regarding the patient; on the other hand, the physician must learn to treat the nurse as an equal with a different task, rather than merely the executor of his demands.

Recognition of the importance of all members of the staff is achieved not just by assertion, but by abolition of the dual chains of command nurses and physicians are governed by. A therapeutic community is maintained through the participation of a team, not only, or even primarily, through the care of the physician, but rather through the counseling and support of all the personnel. A therapeutic community is made possible by a physical environment in which aspects of community living are encouraged for all members—patients, parents, and staff.

Patients can be ministered to in such a community as prize participants, much as children are tended to in a family. The patients are the community's reason for existence, so the community has no self-sustaining rights in the absence of specific patient-directed care goals, even though any given patient is a transient member of the community.

The thesis is that such a therapeutic community accomplishes two things. First, it optimizes the child's quest for normality. Normality does not mean absence of disease or of unpleasant experiences, but an atmosphere in which everything is normal and accepted, whatever has to be accepted. This does not mean that we should generate a "brave new world" in which happiness and virtue are defined as "liking what you've got to do."[22] There is absolutely no demand that a child should like a bone marrow aspiration. Rather the converse, a healthy normal situation should allow him to dislike the dislikable. But a normal situation implies that the necessary is accepted as such.

Second, in a therapeutic community the security each participant has in his role allows that person to become a free human being in interactions with the child-patient. One can befriend a child and yet be a doctor who inflicts pain. Normalcy is perceived both ways. A child with cancer is a child who might die or might live. That is the reality of that child. If he lives, then he should be truly cured. In the final analysis that means that the child is a person in his own right who has the right to live his life as he sees fit within the constraints of the community. He has no obligation to live the way we presuppose he should, especially if we want him to live out our anxieties.

THE THERAPEUTIC COMMUNITY AS A TRAINING GROUND

A therapeutic community is never complete without trainees. They are not a hindrance but an asset. A conceptual division between observing and participating trainees needs to be made. Observing trainees are incidental students who come for a limited time in an assigned role. Participating trainees are those students who learn through the assumption of specific roles in the overall community and therefore need to perform for their own training to be successful. It is clear, then, that in the community there must exist tolerance of ineptness and continuous guidance through new experiences. There should be sufficient mutual respect to allow the inept but capable to learn by experience. There should be enough ego strength to trust experts to express their specific opinion, and yet to be limited by the community to one's own expertise. There should be sufficient respect for the patient and his family to allow his full participation as the primary member of the community. It is necessary to have training and supervision of the inexperienced in interpersonal relationships just as it is necessary to have training in medical lore and nursing skills.

But there is more to training. A common fault of the adult is to become firm in his belief. Training implies teaching beliefs. But transfer of knowledge is never complete, and only by incomplete transfer of knowledge is innovation possible. Assimilation of knowledge is never instantaneous. Only by questioning statements can the students accept. Thus training has a dual role. It allows self-renewal and it demands intellectual honesty. No community could exist without either.

Of course, in a sense the patients fulfill that role also if we just let them. The child who has been diagnosed with cancer has to learn a new reality. He has to question us about what we tell him, and we should be as careful teaching him as we hopefully are teaching the trainees.

WHEN CAN THE TRULY CURED
CHILD BE A CURRENT REALITY?

We have asserted that continuous, complete, unmaintained remissions do not as yet qualify as cures, because a cure means death in old age from unrelated causes. By the same token a truly cured child is that child who becomes an adult able to live to the full extent of his talents. In that sense also we will not know for a long time whether a true cure has been achieved. But just as we may estimate, from the concept of periods of risk, that cures have been achieved biologically long before death, so we can extrapolate from the day-to-day mental growth of the child what the utilization of his potential really is. In fact, it is easier to estimate for child development than for longevity, since educational research has given us many norms against which to measure visual-motor and cognitive development. We have thus a unique situation, in that we can be warned about those children who are not developing and learning at the rate expected for their potential. We can intervene if there are specific identifiable problems.

However, it must be remembered that specific problems are no different from medical complications. A blood transfusion tides a child over a period of marrow depression as much as remedial reading may bring a delayed subunit of the total achievable skills in line with the remainder. But if the child has repeated delays in acquiring skills and there is no medical reason for these delays, the usual treatment is manipulation of the environment. To use the simplest situation, a teacher will ask for a parent conference when a child starts lagging in a subject. The usual questions range around changes in the home environment: the arrival of a sibling, family strife, unusual financial strain. The good teacher will help the parents to cope with the stress placed on the child. In the analogous situation of the child with cancer, the health care delivery teams like to see themselves in the role of the teacher, but they are actually in the role of the parents. An objective evaluation of the child's performance is needed. This evaluation will have to be matched with the medical evaluation to explain any medically caused developmental delays. The remainder must be due in part to the mental upheaval. It is the medical team who is called in by the mental health team to be asked what the problem is that explains this child's distraction. In contrast to our medical management, we have the opportunity to adjust our treatment of the mental and social health of the child as we go along. Treatment of the total child should therefore be easier than the medical treatment, and true cures can be achieved now.

CONCLUDING REMARKS

It may appear that this chapter has stated in a very laborious way that healthy development of children requires a healthy environment. Many would regard that as a truism. Remember, however, that our current cancer center environment is emphatically not conducive to a healthy development, and that we as cancer-care givers are the last to see that we are lacking. Normal child development suggests that the child made the right choices in his growing process. We must supply a healthy selection of options to allow a choice. We cannot afford to wait until our children are adults, because physical cure is around the corner.

REFERENCES

1. Pinkel, D.: Curability of childhood cancer. J. Am. Med. Assoc. 235:1049, 1976.
2. Thomas, L.: To err is human. New Engl. J. Med. 294:99, 1976.
3. McCarthy, D. G. (ed.): Responsible Stewardship of Human Life. The Catholic Hospital Association, St. Louis, 1976.
4. Black, P. M.: Must physicians treat the "whole man" for proper medical care? The Pharos 39:8, 1976.
5. Callahan, D.: The WHO definition of "Health." The Hastings Center Studies 1:77, 1973.
6. Easson, W. M.: The Dying Child. Charles C Thomas, Springfield, Ill., 1970.
7. Easson, W. M.: The Lazarus syndrome in childhood. Med. Insight 4:47, 1972.
8. Price, R. A., and Jamieson, P. A.: The central nervous system in childhood leukemia. II. Subacute leukoencephalopathy. Cancer 35:306, 1975.
9. Rubinstein, L. J., Herman, M. M., Long, T. F., and Wilbur, J. R.: Disseminated necrotizing leukoencephalopathy: a complication of treated central nervous system leukemia and lymphoma. Cancer 35:291, 1975.
10. Soni, S. S., Marteu, G. W., Pitner, S. E., Duenas, D. A., and Powazek, M.: Effects of central-nervous-system irradiation on neuropsychologic functioning of children with acute lymphocytic leukemia. New Engl. J. Med. 293:113, 1975.
11. van Eys, J., Sullivan, M. P., Sutow, W. W., Fernandez, C., Ayala, A. G., Strong, L. C., Du V. Tapley, N., Young, S. E., and Cangir, A.: Childhood tumors. In: R. L. Clark and C. Howe (eds.), Cancer Patient Care at M. D. Anderson Hospital and Tumor Institute. Year Book, Chicago, 1976, p. 309.
12. van Eys, J.: Supportive care of the child with cancer. Ped. Clin. N. Am. 23:215, 1976.
13. Kierkegaard, S.: The Sickness unto Death (W. Lowrie, transl.). Princeton University Press, Princeton, N. J., 1968.
14. Howell, S. E.: Psychiatric aspects of habilitation. Ped. Clin. N. Am. 20:203, 1973.

15. Shepherd, C. W., Jr.: Childhood chronic illness and visual motor development. Except. Child. 36:39, 1969.
16. van Eys, J.: Caring for the child who might die. In: D. E. Barton (ed.), Care for the Dying. Williams & Wilkins, Baltimore, in press.
17. Kübler-Ross, E.: On Death and Dying. Macmillan, New York, 1969.
18. Branson, R.: Is acceptance a denial of death? Another look at Kübler-Ross. The Christian Century 464, 1975.
19. Committee on Hospital Care: Care of Children in Hospitals. 2nd Ed. American Academy of Pediatrics, Evanston, Ill., 1971.
20. Bergmann, T., and Freud, A.: Children in the Hospital. International Universities Press, New York, 1965.
21. Bettelheim, B.: The Empty Fortress. The Free Press, New York, 1967.
22. Huxley, A.: Brave New World. Harper and Brothers, New York, 1950.

CHAPTER 11

The Expectations, Hopes, and Fears of Parents

GINGER PETERSON
and DON PETERSON

Parents of children with a fatal illness should not have significantly different expectations from those of parents of healthy children. Both still would like their child to be developing, without unnecessary obstacles, toward a fully functioning, productive, independent individual. The hope that the child will fulfill these expectations to the desired degree is threatened by his anticipated death, by treatment of the disease process, and by the resulting disturbance of the family unit.[1,2]

Chinn states that in our American culture, in which the present is subordinated to future goals, youth and youthful vigor are admired and valued.[3] When a child who has everything to live for is found to have a fatal illness, the dreams and ideals of the future are suddenly destroyed. In addition, the family may have a great deal of difficulty making optimal use of the time remaining with the child. Many families in our culture have become so preoccupied with the future that they no longer appreciate the present. Finding richness and satisfaction in the experiences that are here and now may be difficult or even impossible. The added stress of facing death rather than the anticipated pleasures of the future further inhibits the appreciation of the child as he is now.

Futterman and Hoffman have described a number of dilemmas which parents confront in adapting to the fatal illness of their child.[4] Parents need to work out a balance between these apparently conflicting adaptive tasks:

Acknowledging the ultimate loss of the child	Maintaining hope
Attending to the immediate needs of the situation	Planning for the future
Cherishing the child	Allowing him to separate
Expressing disturbing feelings	Maintaining day-to-day functioning
Delegating care of the child to medical personnel	Active personal care
Trusting the physician	Recognizing his limitations
Preparing for the child's death through gradual emotional detachment	Caring for the child

The first dilemma is acknowledging the ultimate loss of the child versus maintaining hope. Kübler-Ross states that the physician should always allow for hope, but she adds that this does not always imply hope for survival.[5] If one looks at the first three stages of anticipatory grief which parents go through—acknowledgment, grieving, reconciliation—one can see how parents go from hope of survival fluctuating with despair, to actual grieving over the anticipated loss of the child, to developing a perspective about the child's anticipated death which preserves the parents' sense of confidence in the worth of the child's life and of life in general.[4,6] Leventhal and Hersh, however, bring out the point that for parents to live with such an illness requires some degree of denial, which is acceptable as long as it does not interfere with the parents' ability to cope with the situation.[7]

The second dilemma is attending to the immediate needs of the situation versus planning for the future. Leventhal and Hersh found that the chronic stress of leukemia can be handled more gracefully and with less pain if the family are helped from the beginning to articulate and come to terms with the disease's impact on their lives.[7] Parents should have as much information about the disease, written as well as verbal, as they wish.[8] Through knowledge parents can begin to regain some meaningful control over their own family's destiny.[4] Furthermore, modifications of the family's schedules, plans, and life-styles become more tolerable. However, parents will still find it very difficult to make long- or short-term plans for the future.[7]

The third dilemma deals with cherishing the child while allowing him to separate. One method of coping with the child is to cater or give him special attention. Most parents feel they should not cater to the child yet feel helpless to change this pattern.

The fourth dilemma, that of expressing disturbing feelings versus maintaining day-to-day functioning, implies the double bind of trying to maintain routine daily lives, discipline, and standards while sometimes feeling the need for the financial and emotional burdens to come to an end. Parents generally strive to prolong life as long as possible; however, they also long to be relieved of their burdens and wish to see their child spared.[4]

The fifth dilemma is delegation of care versus active personal care. The child's primary physician often serves as a major source of support.[4] It is important that the primary physician not desert the patient and his family even when the patient no longer meets the medical need "to cure, to treat, to prolong life."[5] Parental coping can be facilitated by allowing parents to participate in the physical and emotional care of their child, if they are able to cope with the responsibilities. Being able to continue with normal functions of the parental role is essential for a less traumatic experience. Special procedures should be taught to the parents, if they are willing, in order to preserve their parental role. However, once parents have received instructions they should not be abandoned, regardless of their apparent expertise.[1]

The sixth dilemma is trusting the physician while recognizing his limitations. Treatments demand intensive participation and cooperation by the patient and his family; these in turn require that there be absolute trust among all parties.[7] Parents frequently insist that they trust the physician without reservations, yet realize that the physician's efforts to control their child's destiny may ultimately be unsuccessful.[8]

The seventh dilemma is preparing for the child's death through gradual detachment versus caring for the child. Kübler-Ross says that when family members have written a patient off it is almost impossible to get them reinvolved.[5] She also discusses the acceptance stage of anticipatory grief, which means acceptance of the finiteness of oneself. Quality of life is different in this stage. Parents and children learn to enjoy today and not worry too much about tomorrow; at the same time they hope to have a long time to enjoy their type of life.

Each of these dilemmas parents face in adapting to the fatal illness of their child has implications to health professionals. Parents need assistance in working out a balance between these conflicting tasks.

Parents of the fatally ill child also experience a series of crises. Although a crisis is an individual matter, referring to personal emotional responses rather than to the situation itself, knowledge of a child's fatal illness will invariably produce crises in a child-oriented, death-avoidance society like ours.[2] It must be remembered that the outcome of a crisis is not predetermined. Whether a person will emerge stronger or weaker is not necessarily determined by his character but by the kind of help he gets during the crisis. It is during crises that parents of the fatally ill child are particularly susceptible to suggestions. This is when intervention for a healthy resolution is essential.[6, 9, 10]   This does not imply solving parents' problems for them, but it does imply guiding parents to healthy alternatives so that the resolution of the crisis is a growth-promoting experience.

In assisting parents in their growth process of adapting to the fatal illness of their child, health care workers assist in the growth process of the child. In so doing, they help parents see some degree of fulfillment of their desired expectations.

We feel several requirements are essential in health care workers who deal with our child:

1. Competency commensurate to one's position
2. Straightforward interchange about the disease and treatment, and honest disclosure when one has reached the limits of his knowledge or current information
3. Demonstration of a sincere interest in the welfare of our child, regardless of personality differences

REFERENCES

1. Fond, K. I.: Dealing with death and dying through family-centered care. Nursing Clin. N. Am. 7:53, 1972.
2. Mann, S.: Coping with a child's fatal illness. Nursing Clin. N. Am. 9:81, 1974.
3. Chinn, P.: Child Health Maintenance. C. V. Mosby, St. Louis, 1974.
4. Futterman, E., and Hoffman, I.: Crises and adaptation in families of fatally ill children. In: The Child in His Family. John Wiley & Sons, New York, 1973.
5. Kübler-Ross, E.: Coping with Death and Dying. Series of five tapes. 1973.
6. Parad, H. J.: Crisis Intervention: Selected Readings. Family Service Association of America, New York, 1965.
7. Leventhal, B., and Hersh, S.: Modern treatment of childhood leukemia: the patient and his family. Nursing Digest 3:12, 1975.
8. Evans, A.: Practical care for the family of a child with cancer. Cancer 35:871, 1975.
9. Aguilera, D., Messick, J., and Farrell, M.: Crisis Intervention: Theory and Methodology. C. V. Mosby, St. Louis, 1970.
10. Cadden, V.: Crisis in the Family. National Research Bureau, Chicago.

SECTION V

The Insights of the Participants

CHAPTER 12

Introduction

JAN VAN EYS

The discussions held among the various participants brought to light a surprising number of common concerns, shared anxieties, and previously unvoiced aspirations. The leaders of the sessions needed only to be facilitators. The spirit of the meetings was such that little prompting or guiding was necessary. At all times three groups gathered with two discussion leaders. Discussions were held after each of the three sessions. The discussion leaders rotated, so no team was alike in any group.

It was, of course, inevitable that the discussion leaders heard and assimilated the interchanges in various ways. The ideas discussed sent their own thoughts in various directions, and the summary papers reflect this. Some discussion leaders were awed and inspired by the interchanges; their papers are faithful summaries, brightened by their delight. Others had their own concepts strengthened, and they described the sessions as if they were one step removed. What may seem repetition at first glance was often recorded as different percepts. The groups struggled with the same problems and contributed complementary insights.

It would be surprising if not one among the participants asks, "Is that what we said?" Maybe it was not what was said, but only what was heard. On the other hand, it may indeed have been said, but not understood by all participants. In any discussion there will always be thoughts expressed that have no impact, while passing remarks may touch off strong reactions. But such is the strength of dialogue. The workshop did not solve all problems, but it did remove perception barriers. The following pages demonstrate the remarkable degree to which this occurred.

CHAPTER 13

Reflections of a Psychologist

RICHARD BENTON

THE CONFLICT BETWEEN THE PATIENT AND THE
DEMANDS IMPOSED BY INSTITUTION AND RESEARCH

This section could equally well be labeled "the conflict between individualism and collectivism" or "group processing." We in the United States, perhaps more than in any other nation, worship institutions. Institutions provide us with a seemingly efficient way of transacting business. They give us a means of identifying the steps through which we may proceed in a given transaction, and thus help minimize anxiety. We treat anxiety as a fearful illness, and we attempt to be strictly logical. But in institutions in which the healing arts are practiced, anxiety is high even when institutional rules are orderly. Of course, there are the "free spirits" who become anxious when rules are imposed. But there are always emotions with which one has to contend: the very human side of people with illness.

Under stress, people often reach for a response to help them through the period. Often their reactions do not follow patterns consistent with the logical rules of the institution. The person under stress may be unable to see the rationale for the rules. The assigned bureaucrat, in turn, may become frustrated and react toward the transgressor of rules as though he were a saboteur. These transactions simply exacerbate the situation: neither side is able to read the other's position. The hospital employee has a vested interest, but so does the patient or relative. Sometimes neither party is able to understand the other, so the patient ends up "going along." The patient must react emotionally to rules and procedures he cannot understand. Without some degree of structure he reacts with superstition, anger, submissiveness, perplexity, or withdrawal. In some instances, he may attempt to prepare himself by study.

Many of these conflicts are not obvious to the patient who is unable to verbalize them. For example, patients and families have surgical procedures described to them in substantial detail. But many patients have verbal fluencies within the dull normal or even borderline mentally retarded ranges. Under such circumstances, while it might appear that the rights of the individual have been protected through informed consent, from another point of view it may be argued that no adequate explanation was given. In one case which I recall, the gravity of an operation was being explained to a patient's family in an attempt to obtain their understanding and consent. After considerable discussion one of the relatives asked, "How long will the scar be?" The reply was that the scar would be approximately twelve to fourteen inches long, a length which the doctor demonstrated. At that point the relatives exclaimed, "My goodness, that is indeed a serious operation!" They seemed immediately to grasp the gravity of the procedure. Different cultural and ethnic groups place different importance on procedures performed on specific body sites. Such subtle distinctions may influence understanding of related explanations. Informed consent could be carried to the point at which progress within human medical science would be curtailed. Thus, some decisions must be made without fully informed consent.

In our discussion groups one participant, a member of a research review committee, said his committee had much difficulty evaluating the informed consent forms that must be delivered to participating patients. At present it has no effective way of monitoring presentation and/or level of communication to participating patients. The existence of such a committee, however, is a decided improvement over prior procedures for conducting research, which had no requirements for informed consent. The group endorsed a reasonable level of informed consent.

Hospitals are businesses even when not for profit. This causes a demand for self-sufficiency and hence a vested interest. A dimension of vested interest is expressed by the term "self-serving," which is frequently treated, especially by those in the helping profession, as a dirty word. Yet we may all be accused of being self-serving in that we attempt to promote, maintain, or secure our own interests. If hospital employees want someone around to help, then they are serving their own needs. On an institutional level, departments as well as individuals become self-serving through efforts to obtain and to balance tenure and benefit. Some institutions have been accused of withholding curative processes as a self-serving tactic. It is unlikely that such practices have actually occurred in recent times.

Two other topics were discussed relating to hospitals and patient needs. These were system problems and delegation of power. System problems discussions revolved around rules and their flexibility or inflexibility. Frequently an institution has no procedures to review rules, and so they accumulate and are never updated. As this occurs, people outside of patient contact areas come to administer rules in an impersonal, bureaucratic, and even cumbersome fashion. Frequently rules lose their purpose and hinder rather than assist patient flow and treatment procedures.

During discussion of delegation of power, it was suggested that institutions act on the public level as though power struggles and personalities did not exist. This is, of course, a fallacy since these struggles and personalities in many ways flavor the administrative structures of institutions. In many, if not most, instances power is not spoken of openly, but it still exists. It is usually detected through the level and mode of delegation of responsibilities. Frequently failure to delegate power is excused because of lack of knowledge when actually it is a protective strategy of individuals. While there is general agreement that such motives operate, they are rarely voiced. Those in positions of power rarely grant permission to disclose.

THE CONFLICT BETWEEN THE PERSONAL NEEDS OF THE STAFF AND THE IDEAL OF HUMANE PATIENT TREATMENT

Discussion of topics relating to the conflict between the personal needs of the staff and the ideal of humane patient treatment centered around several topics. The first was the concept of meaningful treatment by the physician and treatment staffs. Several physicians admitted that they frequently approach the patient as a disease, minimizing the human aspects of the disease. They address the mechanical and technical procedures used to remedy the illness, and develop an "acute" cure attitude that does not result in a program dedicated to the treatment of the whole person. They look at the disease that can be most readily treated with prevailing techniques to give the most dramatic response. This attitude minimizes futuristic outcomes and the larger problems that are more difficult to contend with.

Still, many treatment procedures ameliorate the bodily insult and allow the individual to continue living, though altered in some degree. The resulting difference in life-style is frequently denied or ignored, even though such alterations ripple through the individual family and community. This rippling creates emotional reactions that persist throughout the course of the disease. Especially marked and dramatic changes may lead to divorce, individual alienation, and emotional stress. Thus, disease has not only physical dimensions but also metaphysical dimensions. Although the latter dimensions are less tangible and certainly less directly observable, they are clearly felt. Those who deal with physical problems should also deal with these sometimes more difficult and frustrating problems.

The consequences of the treatment regimen itself, in terms of cosmetic results and quality of survival, were also discussed. Frequently the physician confers with the patient, describing visible consequences of the procedure, instilling confidence in the patient, and helping him to prepare for these changes. Quality of survival is a more nebulous, longer-ranged concept that is less frequently dealt with on an adequate basis by physician and patient. This is due at least in part to the fuzziness of the term. Physicians typically avoid terms which are poorly defined and which cannot be adequately demonstrated. (Of course, omission is one way of dealing with an issue.) Quality of survival raises the question whether or not the end justifies the means in treatment procedure. Sometimes treatment procedures are withheld to avoid the appearance of the means justifying the end. However, withholding a certain treatment procedure is in itself a treatment procedure.

Finally the views of living and dying are often difficult for patient, family, and physician. The problems relating to a child dying before adulthood were discussed. In our culture the death of children stirs substantial guilt feelings among physicians who treat the children, as well as among parents and relatives who are unable to bestow adulthood upon the child. A substantial part of our lives is devoted to training for adulthood. The child who dies is prevented from attaining this end. Some children are regarded as sources of immortality by their parents. Being unable to see that a child achieves adulthood frequently results in anxiety. In earlier days families were larger and children died more frequently; this may have diminished some of the fear which is seen today in smaller families.

THE TRULY CURED CHILD

Topics relating to the discussion of the truly cured child included the definition of "cured" and the conflicts between the physician's view of this term and the expectations of parents and patients. Individuals often conceive of cure in an acute sense. This does not treat the patient as a whole, nor does it view life in long range terms. Some suggested that there is no such thing as a cure, that the term is a fallacy representing our wish to deny death. In a sense, curative procedures only postpone death by diminishing the acute insult on a particular occasion.

The participants again addressed the question of the meaning of cancer and death. The general consensus was that, in many patient populations, cancer does mean death. Indeed, this appears to be the general population's emotional understanding of the term. It also came to light that many nursing staff members identify cancer with death. They have difficulty convincing patients that cancer can be cured since many hospital beds are filled with dying people. Thus, many hospital ward nurses become deaf to the optimistic statistics frequently quoted by hospital physicians and begin to react fearfully themselves.

CHAPTER 14

A Community in Conversation

MARGARET BUCHORN

Before beginning the first group, I felt it important to clarify a possible misunderstanding in the invitational letter. I believe that many of the problems which arise among staff members anywhere are due to faulty communications. The day before the workshop began, a parent who planned to participate interpreted a statement in the letter to mean that current problems in pediatrics were not to be discussed. At my request one of the group read the letter and found this statement was indeed ambiguous.* I felt it important to establish from the beginning that our purpose was not to be a "bitching" group, nor were we gathered to evaluate the functioning of particular pediatric staff members. However, we could recognize weaknesses and deficiencies only by discussing them. This was the only way we could become aware of needed improvements. Our goal was better functioning, better participation, and a more open facility. At times we would need to discuss our weaknesses in order to determine how we could improve. Therefore, everyone needed to understand that full participation on their part involved critical as well as laudatory statements.

THE RIGHTS OF THE CHILD AND
THE PROBLEMS OF THE INSTITUTION

Dr. Richie's presentation raised the issue of children's rights. Our society is just beginning to look at the problem of groups without civil rights, for whom others make basic decisions. Institutions established to protect the child, while benevolent in intent, are being questioned. Such institutions may be more harmful than helpful to the best interests of the child. It is in this area that I have always perceived pediatrics as being uniquely difficult and painful; there is a critical difference between making permanent or life-threatening decisions for oneself and making them for one's child. The fact that a small child lacks competence because of his inadequate life experience cannot be denied. The group discussed measures of competence and decided that even preschool children could be usefully included in the process of decision making, although not made responsible for the decisions. The parent was cited as the benevolent actor for the child, in turn raising the

---

*The statement read: "Our goal is not so much to discuss existing problems. Rather it will focus on how to avoid future problems and to come to an understanding of what our roles are in achieving a truly cured child."

question of the parent's competence to make decisions on the basis of highly technical, specialized information. This led naturally into a discussion of health care personnel's responsibility to share information with parents. We must guard against the frequent practice of benevolent physicians deciding for the parent, who is presumably deciding for the child, because they perceive both as incompetent. Competence in medical consent is actually involved much less with technical knowledge than with what a particular family is willing to endure or impose upon its child for a problematical outcome. This is a moral, philosophical decision, not a medical one.

One parent brought up the moral issue of a physician influencing an ill person whose judgment may be affected both by his illness and by his trusting relationship with the doctor. The competence of an ill person differs from that of a healthy person. This parent also focused on the conflict that occurs when the attending physician presents one treatment as preferable to another. If the parent refuses the treatment the physician prefers, he appears unwilling to do what is best for his child. A physician who returned to M. D. Anderson after twenty-five years spoke of his awe not only at the technical advances but also at the complexity and size of the institution. He was amazed at the infinite patience of people who come to the hospital.The patients' obviously very high expectations made him feel very inadequate. The possibility of having an ombudsman, someone available to the patient and his family at all times as their advocate, was discussed. The present practice in the Department of Pediatrics of assigning a staff physician as the patient's private physician was seen as a move in this direction.

A short discussion followed on the conflict between patient care and education and research interest. The increased turnover of physicians in training often makes it necessary for families to adjust to a new person on each return visit. Since parents know that these physicians are being trained, they sometimes feel that inadequately trained people are dealing with their children. The fact that young trainees are often better able to deal with emergency situations was recognized. However, the point at issue is the extra burden placed upon families who must relate to different physicians at each monthly visit. The emotional difficulties involved were discussed.

One of the parents noted that we had asked that she speak with absolute frankness. She then stated that she would never admit her child without being present nor would she allow procedures to be done except in her presence. She is herself a health care professional and is aware that people have to learn; however, she thinks that many young physicians do not realize when they should call in someone more experienced. The appropriateness of the parent's being present as the protector of his child was validated. There was also discussion of the parent being the person most aware of the child's tolerance of particular procedures.

The importance of physicians' learning to admit that they cannot do a particular thing at a particular time was stressed. The myth that physicians have to be supermen needs to be dealt with openly. The importance of information being given to patients at all times before procedures are initiated was stressed by both the administrators and the parents in the group. Anytime someone understands the necessity for a procedure being done, he is much more likely not only to accept but to facilitate the procedure. Limitations imposed both by the number of patients and by the severity of their illness are one reason for the curtailment of information giving and other interrelations between staff and patients. An excellent case was made that both physicians and laboratory personnel are overburdened. One physician described how he is subordinating his private life in order to better serve his patients. He is in a special situation because he has no family responsibilities at this time. One participant asked how adequately we serve the needs of others when we do so at the expense of our own needs. The group generally felt that this is not a healthy situation for anyone to remain in for any period of time.

Considerable discussion centered around particular problems posed by parents' being present while children were being treated. The distinction was made between what is better for the child and what is easier for the staff. It is always easier for the staff to do a particular procedure without parents. However, if the parents are not dealt with they could project their own fears onto the child. Again, the necessity for parental involvement on as many levels as possible was emphasized.

We next discussed the fact that people who work in situations that require dealing with pain and distress protect themselves by falling back on policies and routines. That all people who work in such situations must constantly remind themselves how it feels to be on the other side of the desk or needle cannot be overemphasized.

Some of the infuriating delays at M. D. Anderson are related to the need for a person to bring the medical chart. This is one effect of the institution's policy that everyone has access to the patient's chart except the patient. The oft-repeated pros and cons of allowing patients to read their medical charts were discussed. Allowing patients to read their own records, particularly comments involving family problems or social information, was characterized by one physician as dangerous. He was questioned, "Dangerous to whom?" We seem to be protecting ourselves rather than the patient. Hospital records are available to everyone in the institution and much of the information in them is handled in a very unprofessional fashion. We are all aware of this. Certainly the person about whom the information is written is already aware of his own life situation or family problems. The staff's preventing a patient from reading his record is comparable to a parent's withholding a child's correct diagnosis to protect the child. One parent commented that when he is *not* given information he becomes upset and questions and wonders about the adequacy of treatment.

The group discussed the subject of parents who are left out because of their inability to speak English. The institution appears remiss in not having enough competent interpreters. I consider the use of other parents as interpreters bad practice. Translating one language into another is a skill not everyone has. Moreover, using another patient as an interpreter destroys the confidentiality of the situation and imposes upon the patient serving as interpreter. This is often done through necessity, but it should not be condoned. One physician spoke of his frustration when he is not able to adequately communicate with a family especially when their child becomes critically ill. He was acutely aware of the additional anxiety involved for the parent at such a time. A parent spoke of a time when another parent serving as an interpreter had to neglect her own child to meet the hospital's need. The comment was made that the hospital administration should recognize Texas is a bilingual state. A further comment was that parents who are not being communicated with are accustomed to having their feelings ignored, and so administrative powers have assumed that this is no problem. Some patients and families elect to put themselves in an interpretive role because they allay their own feelings of helplessness.

One mother said that, in spite of all the hospital defects, when her child must be admitted to the pediatric floor she feels that the whole family is admitted. She sees this as an unifying, supportive approach. Someone wondered if all of the difficulties we were talking about that morning were not related to faulty communication between patients and staff or between staff and staff. While using difficulty in communication to explain everything may be overly facile, there is some accuracy in the comment. The example of a Vietnamese patient with whom no one on the staff could communicate verbally and yet with whom many staff members communicated on an emotional level was cited. The problem is that we communicate at all times with people, whether we verbalize or not, and we get into difficulties when we communicate one message verbally and another nonverbally. The important factor is what underlies the communication we are giving patients. If we are willing to be involved, our commitment to the worth and dignity of the patient will be communicated. An excellent example was offered by a lab technician who told how she tries to train new personnel to wake up patients at 7:00 A.M. to draw blood. Her own conviction that patients have a right to be awakened gently, to refuse treatment, and to be grumpy obviously is conveyed to the patients as respect.

The point was made that many patients take out on the hospital personnel their fear and anger over what must be done to them. An additional point was made that many times patients are fearful of directly expressing these feelings to their physicians; instead, they express them to technicians and nurses. Several witnessed to the importance of personnel's spending enough time with the patient. The fact that spending time with the patient in a moment of crisis or early in the relationship often saves time later on is not perceived by enough of us.

THE FEELINGS OF THE STAFF

The Saturday afternoon session dealt more specifically with "bricks and mortar." Some of the discussion arose directly out of the paper I had presented. The nursing staff was particularly concerned that staff and other parents are critical of mothers' going out, leaving their child during the hospital stay, even though the hospital itself, through the Social Service and Volunteer Departments, encourages this. This discussion was enlarged with some consideration of the staff's role with patients. As our area of concern is not really the patient's or the parent's life-style, it is important that we not be judgmental. However, open disapproval is often easier to handle than "double messages." Those of us in the helping professions should acknowledge openly when we disapprove of others.

The mothers or other caregivers who have been at their child's bedside in long vigils greatly need some respite. Many need considerable encouragement before they will allow themselves to leave the child.

This is beneficial for the mother, for the child, and for the staff. I don't think there is any real argument about this. These respites need to be fostered, but both mothers and staff resist them. This resistance cannot be handled by staff in an authoritative way without gross infringement of the patient's rights. We were talking about people's acceptance of people different from themselves. Learning acceptance has to be a constant, ongoing educational process.

A recent example of hard-to-accept behavior occurred with the admission of a youngster whose vocabulary was offensive to many on the staff, including the department head. This very young child responded with four-letter words to any attempt to treat him. The child had learned this behavior from the adults around him, who used the same vocabulary and felt no need to correct him. This made difficulties for those staff members unaccustomed to being greeted in this fashion. It was well that everyone recognized that this was difficult. On the other hand, what did this child's vocabulary have to do with his medical care or treatment?

A physical therapist described a highly intelligent child who handled much of his anxiety and energies by going on rounds with the physicians. The physical therapists were amazed when they were written a "consult" to exercise this patient one hour. Obviously what they were being asked to do was to help control the child's behavior, not provide physical therapy. While recreational therapy with children has a place in overall hospital care, it is not the function of the Physical Therapy Department to serve this purpose.

We next discussed factors that motivate the staff. As mentioned earlier, a consulting physician had commented in the morning session that he was constantly impressed that patients at M. D. Anderson tolerate much more waiting and physical inconvenience than they would anywhere else. He attributed this to two factors: patients come to M. D. Anderson with such terrible problems, and they are coming to "mecca" and expect miracles. Many patients come to M. D. Anderson after having been actively discouraged by their local physician and others. When they are met with hope at the treatment facility, they respond with tremendous elation and relief. Everyone who is dealing with such patients has to be careful not to build this into unrealistic optimism. It is always a temptation for a helping professional to be a "rescuer."

Anyone who works in a cancer center is constantly asked by colleagues and friends how they can endure it. The personality traits which lead professionals into choosing cancer patients have been considered very little. My experience is that personnel generally either leave M. D. Anderson very rapidly or settle down for a long stay. Those unable to tolerate cancer patients are well advised to leave quickly, both for themselves and for the patients. This led into a spirited discussion of how an institution could and should support the emotional needs of its staff. The consensus was that a planned orientation to cancer patients, with emphasis on emotional problem areas such as disfigurement, length of illness, and death, is indicated. Ongoing, built-in mental health facilities for staff are badly needed. Also, outside stimulation for all of the professional staff, with encouragement for continuing education and professional growth, was seen as an effective way of combatting routinized stress. M. D. Anderson, with its emphasis on the importance of the medical staff at the expense of the other professional personnel, is sadly lacking in these activities. The Nursing Department is perhaps the most supportive and encouraging of the nonphysician staff.

THE CONCEPT OF CURE

The Sunday afternoon discussion was the liveliest of the three. The group was sparked by Dr. van Eys' concept of cure and by the Petersons' view that parents are not primarily interested in prolonging their child's life but rather in making the best use of that life. I had some initial concern that this group was too large for satisfactory discussion. While there were many auditors, it was heartening to hear from some subsequently that they had gained much from the discussion.

The concept of cure and its cost seemed particularly troubling to many physicians. I quoted a physician I had heard that morning on television explain that he removed disease, only Jesus cured. This concept seemed more comfortable for some of the physicians. One immediately introduced his concern that many colleagues do not come to terms with the reality of the naturalness and inevitability of death. Our culture wishes to deny this natural process, and this denial can be seen in the current medical zeal to conquer all. I mentioned another concept of death as not only natural, but necessary, to life. One could speculate on the desirability of immortality in the form of life which we presently know. How many of us would elect endless days in a nursing home, for instance? The frightening cost to the patient and his family of current methods of prolongation of a child's life was approached from different points. The lessened cognitive functions and disfigurement often accompanying the "cure" were perceived by many as too great a cost.

I cited a recent conversation with the grandmother of a fourteen-year-old boy, in which she stated that, could the family really have understood all of the implications four years ago, they probably would have chosen death. She felt certain that the patient himself would have so chosen. The reality, as reiterated throughout this discussion by one mother, is that parents at the time have no choice. Hindsight is always a great enlightener. At the time of the decision a parent can only ask for life. While not disputing this, some physicians revealed not only their own conflicts in participating in some of these "cures," but their regret at not making greater efforts to prepare parents or help them consider alternatives. Most felt that the weight of the institution, research considerations, and so forth, were so heavily placed upon "cure" or "progress" that not enough time and thought were given to the possible negative aspects. One physician commented that medical cure is certainly not the only factor to be considered.

One of the group who teaches handicapped children protested some of these assertions, stating that in her experience no handicapped child would prefer death. Being handicapped by an accident of birth or an external happening is very different from being handicapped as a result of a deliberate, thoughtful decision. This difference is felt by the child patient, the parent, and the physician who is influencing or at least implementing the decision. The later responsibility and blame, if any, are of a very different nature. Our limitations in perceiving another life from our own experience are illuminating. I am reminded of a two-and-a-half-year-old who was angry that her colostomy had been repaired. Her earliest memories were of painless stool activity and a distinctive "button"; her normality was not that of the adults who were so happy at being able to restore her. We should be aware of what the Petersons presented so forcibly—the perceived crisis may not be truly serious.

A parent spoke movingly of her conviction that her son lived longer than appropriate for his own well-being in a successful effort to give the family time to work out their own adjustment and resolution. The commonly experienced but often denied fact is that many patients choose their own time of death by either prolonging their lives for others or refusing to actively cooperate because of lack of interest. The superiority of the spirit over the body is something modern man, enamored of his technological mastery, needs to be reminded of. How protective dying persons are of their families and staff is often ignored but needs recognition. We often assume that only adults protect children. I can cite many instances in which children confided their recognition of their parents' or their doctors' inability to deal with their death. This is another reason why it is imperative that an adequate pediatric service include a variety of adults capable of being a "friend" such as Dr. van Eys defined.

The Petersons had suggested that caring personnel are the best help and support of parents. This was a flattering and hopeful concept to me as a professional engaged in helping people learn to cope, but I questioned it. However, parents in the group validated this position without reservation; they felt that many times the supportive, understanding atmosphere of the cancer center was much more valuable than the actual treatment offered. One parent added that the day she saw the fewest physicians was the day her child died. She knew that the physicians had nothing medically to offer, but she needed their human concern and sympathy. We agreed that many times physicians sell themselves short in failing to recognize that the greatest gift one human being can give another is his concerned presence.

The group preferred to discuss absence of disease rather than cure. They preferred to consider an integrated, well rounded life above the conquest of cancer. They hoped for a return to the recognition of the human and spiritual values which at times seem forgotten in our quest for scientific advancement.

CHAPTER 15

The Therapeutic Community: A Reflective Discussion

JOSEPH F. O'DONNELL

The use of language, a philosophy of care, an anxious and urgent plea for openness and candor, and a feeling that we have made some progress toward the formation of a truly therapeutic community—these became the primary foci of a lively series of discussions.

COMMUNICATION

"Maybe we shouldn't use the word," reflected one physician. The use of the term "cancer" seems to produce, in medical and nonmedical personnel alike, the automatic reaction of terminality. "Cancer" means "death," it is as simple as that. "When I was eleven, a year after my diagnosis," commented a patient (now twenty-one), "I looked up the term 'Hodgkin's disease' in the dictionary; it said, 'Cancer, eventually fatal.' " (Later on he could laugh to his mother that the dictionary was wrong.) Common knowledge about cancer still assumes that the patient will die within a short time. At senior prom, a high school counselor asked a patient (then diagnosed for six years) how long he would live, and if he was enjoying his last fling.

Medical personnel tend to use individual terms such as "Hodgkin's disease," "Wilms' tumor," and "acute leukemia" because there has been real success in the treatment of these diseases. The terms "lymphoma" and "neuroblastoma" are used much less often because there has been relatively little success in these areas.

With the progress in cancer treatment, commented a physician, "cancer is a chronic rather than a special disease." We ought to look upon it as we do diabetes mellitus, kidney disease, or even mental retardation. But this view might bring resistance from the "cancer establishment." A large portion of research funds come from the Department of Health, Education, and Welfare. If cancer ceases to be a "special interest," such funds could be directed to other, apparently more pressing needs. More money is spent on cancer research than on sudden infant mortality and premature birth, both of which kill more children than cancer in the first year of life. We might be "stuck with present remedies and their refinements, rather than moving forward toward full cure."

We constantly need to look at ourselves. Throughout the discussions, efforts made to focus on reasons and feelings within the participants were often redirected away from them. Nowhere did this become more clear than in the area of communication.

While noting that each child, and each parent, is different, the patients made an overwhelmingly clear plea for more information. "When I was ten," one young man said, "I thought it [Hodgkin's disease] was just like having a sore throat, appendectomy, or a broken leg. When it finally got to me that it would always be there, then I wanted to know everything." The parents of this patient chose not to tell him for several years that he had cancer, but he learned it by himself, by reading and listening. Another patient omitted listing her cancer as a "serious disease" on her university application blank because such a concept had never occurred to her. In the clinic one day, an eleven-year-old was overheard telling a five-year-old that "there was no cure for his cancer, but there were lots of treatments." Both children seemed comfortable with this communication.

Two important factors came to light here: the question as to who is actually being protected by the withholding of information, and the validity of the assumption that older children (eleven to thirteen years old) who do not ask do not want to know the truth of their disease. The feelings of the physician or of the parents may impede the flow of knowledge. One physician said that no pediatric patient had ever asked for information. But very often the questions are asked indirectly. Patients hesitate for a number of reasons: already knowing the answer, being afraid to hear, or not trusting anyone enough to ask. It is most difficult to *hear* the feelings of the patient when he asks, especially if our own defenses interfere with the process of communication. The physician must create a climate in which information may be requested and shared.

The process of communication ought to begin on the first day of admission, but the newness, the fear and stress, bewilderment and awe, make this almost impossible for patients. There are so many people, both staff and patients, so many things to do and places to be, and often a sense of loss due to the very size of the building (or the size of Houston, for out-of-towners). "I listened hard," said a parent, "but when I got home and tried to explain it to someone else, I found that I had barely grasped anything."

Thus the timeliness of giving information is particularly important. Knowing the patient and the family is an obligation incumbent upon the primary physician, even if much of the actual sharing will be done by the resident and intern. Each physician must be careful not to presume that he knows better than the patient what the patient can handle. "It is much more difficult when you do not know what is going on. I don't even mind a new protocol or experiment as long as you tell me what you are doing," said one patient. Another patient added, "If you told me that I had two months to live, I would begin to deal with it; however, if I found it out by myself, wow!" When a doctor cautioned about the possibility of being wrong, a patient quickly replied, "I wouldn't mind!"

The patients and parents present at the discussion were quite vocal and obviously more capable of handling information than many others not present. There are angry and terrified parents, parents hesitant or unable to ask (and physicians hesitant or unable to tell). A very debilitating "conspiracy of silence" can result. "It is best to know," said a patient, "because it generates honesty and confidence." The physician should probe for questions, even ask, "Do you want to know what you have?" Telling the patient that there is no answer right now is itself an acceptable answer.

Much information is passed on the wards and in the clinic. Patients and families compare medications and treatments, assess the staff members, and form their own close-knit community over which the physician has little control. A good deal of misinformation is shared also. Some parents caution newcomers not to compare. Some parents ask nothing. Others ask the wrong people, either because they want only answers they will like or because a particular person is open and trusting. Nonmedical personnel receive many questions regarding medical care.

The institution involves many people working together and influencing the patient and the family. This may be threatening to the physician who wants absolute control over the situation. Yet he sees the patient perhaps thirty minutes a day, while the nursing personnel are there for eight hours, teachers for six, other professionals for shorter periods, and the captive parent(s) all day. "The doctors come, write orders, and leave," remarked a patient. "The rest of the staff is there all the time. So I always say, 'I'm fine,' to the doctor; then the rest find out what is really wrong with me." Patients and families realize the pressure of time on the physician and respond accordingly, even if this impedes the flow of reliable information.

The absence of communication was illustrated by a long discussion of the medical chart. One physician defended the ownership of the chart by the hospital, citing the legal implications, need for confidentiality, and funding and accreditation requirements. Parents pressed only for the information in the chart, not the chart itself. Almost everyone in the hospital except the patient himself can read the chart. He is protected from it even to the point of severe inconvenience, having to wait often unreasonably long for a patient transportation clerk to carry his chart from one place to the next. The chart became a symbol of the plea for more information.

Soon after first admission, both medical and emotional ties to the institution and its personnel develop and become a source of tension. Patients and families often refer to all places other than M. D. Anderson as "the outside." There is a sense of security and personal reliance on the larger, more specialized institution. "They know what they are doing," said a patient who admitted never going to his local physician for anything. When it was suggested that M. D. Anderson was a sort of "medical mecca," all the patients and parents responded most affirmatively. "They gave me my son for a year and a half," said one mother with a burst of emotion. The true professional is at M. D. Anderson; the local physician is just not as good. This is unfair, but it is a real feeling.

The local physician is very important. He first sees the patient and makes the referral. He may react by getting excited about the disease, by reading and becoming informed, or by feeling that he will never see that disease again and not delve into it at all. The possibility of professional jealousy exists. Sometimes, when a child goes home, the parent informs the physician at home of the nature of the home protocol, the requirements for its administration, and the side effects anticipated. The parent may know more about the disease or treatment than the doctor. Efforts have been made to improve communication with the local physician. A recent symposium received a poor response, and more needs to be done.

Simultaneously, the larger institution may foster a feeling of total reliance on itself. "It is more practical to have them here," said one physician. "Indeed," said another, "I'm always happier when the patient is from Houston." A third admitted that patients are often kept in the hospital for longer periods than really necessary and are frequently brought back to the hospital sooner because of a lack of confidence in the physician at home.

These ties to the institution are essential to long-term follow-up and continued research. Because cancer affects growing tissue in a growing organism, doctors need to have cumulative results and to know the total period of risk. This is especially true for pediatric cancer.

NORMALCY

M. D. Anderson has been referred to as "one huge therapy group." Much of the needed care is not medical. Physical, psychological, financial, and social factors have to be integrated into the community life of the patient if there is to be any semblance of a normal atmosphere. The exceptional nature of the group itself, on the ward or in the clinic, is significant to the formation of this milieu. There is a sophistication among the patients, and often their families, that includes such "hospital wisdom" as what to ask and what not to ask, whom to ask and whom to avoid, and a generous knowledge of the protocols and equipment themselves.

Particularly important in the formation of the community is the tendency of patient and parent to choose a friend. While this is often a staff member, it can be another patient or parent. Choosing a friend always involves a risk, but that in itself is a basic element in any community. A sensitive staff member will realize, for example, that it is possible and permissible to be both physician *and* friend to the patient.

The abilities of the group and the presence of a friend or confidant can help to alleviate the visible stress of the ward environment. There is continual confrontation with reality in the presence of death about every ten days. No one is unaffected by this. Even visiting physicians from other hospitals have a most difficult time because they are accustomed to seeing children die only in premature nurseries. The many little things can hamper the effort to build a community—the crowding in rooms, the lack of privacy (sometimes even for death), the shortage of staff (forcing some parents to assume more patient care than they might care to have, and creating tension if another parent chooses to leave the ward for any reason), the lack of space to talk or to cry, the absence of even basic facilities (such as cooking and laundry) for the nonpatient "inmates" of the ward.

The presence of siblings at home increases the frustration of both patients and parents. It is simply not possible to do justice to both the sick child in the hospital and the well child or children (who may at times wish to be sick in order to get some attention) at home. Stress can grow between spouses who are separated by reason of the illness, and marital difficulties that may have preceded the sickness are compounded by the separation. Only about ten percent of the patients are from the Houston area, and fully one-third are from outside the United States.

In the midst of this, there is the need to create an atmosphere in which a child can continue to grow and develop normally, despite his illness. He cannot be sick for three years and then function fully when he leaves the hospital if he has not continued his emotional and educational growth during the intervening period. It is not possible to play "catch-up ball." It is difficult not to cater to a sick child, even when knowing that he can manipulate his entire environment. "It was most difficult to insist that he do schoolwork, to prod and prod," said a mother, "but if we had let him go at age ten and not do the work, we feel that he would never have reached this far." (The patient is now twenty-one and a college student.) The presence of any limitations due to the sickness ought not to affect the child any more than other limitations of life affect a healthy child.

COMMUNITY

The opportunity exists today to develop a truly positive community of cancer cure and care, with all its attendant risks. We can be very hopeful, and we need to examine our feelings. Can we overcome the frustrations of the system, and our own as well, and look to each day with an attitude of openness and confidence that cancer no longer means death, and that a normal life is within reach of many of our patients? We should not wait for a better environment before changing things for the better. For every patient we send out cured, there are always two more waiting to come in. The new facilities will ease some things, but they may also increase tensions in other areas. The future is now, for us.

We need to look within ourselves. We need trust, and we need to justify that trust. We need to admit that not all members of the staff will do equally well, that students and young professionals may on occasion be painfully inept, and that each of us may not always put his best foot forward. We need to speak to the feelings of all who come on the ward—to see, for example, how the laboratory technician feels about always having to be the bad person who sticks the patient. We need to shorten the long hours of waiting, to simplify procedures as much as possible, to meet the individual needs of patient and family, as well as those of the staff and the institution.

Indeed, we need to allow for our own *humanness*. A sense of the ultimate reality becomes a part of the "normalcy" mentioned earlier. A mother spoke of going along fine for several years, and then of having all the old fears return in an instant when her son was asked to undergo another biopsy. It is a fact that each of us must die. But our lives are not lived in constant fluctuation between imminent death and cure. We do not know what will happen. We *do* know that great progress has been made in the treatment of this disease. We must encourage patients and parents to live life now, to the fullest extent possible. The alternative is a child whose growth and training have been stifled during the time he has been sick; he falls behind in every way. In addition, failure to live life now may trigger the emergence of the "Lazarus syndrome," a condition in which the family is not emotionally ready to handle this child who has "returned from the dead."

"People get well by medical care and by people caring," said a psychologist, "and the question is 'How much will you be a person?'" Some relationship to the patient is established by each person in the community, either simply by doing his professional best or by a deeper and more involved concern for the whole person. If we reach for this, we will achieve our goal of a therapeutic community. The cure of cancer is here for many of our patients; the challenge for each of us is to deal with this great reality.

CHAPTER 16

What Are We All About?

TERRY RULFS

On Saturday and Sunday, March 13th and 14th, Pediatrics did indeed look at itself, inside, outside, and creatively. With a diversified group consisting of doctors, nurses, psychologists, technicians, therapists, chaplains, parents of patients, patients, and others I am sure I have not recalled, we were able to combine our ideas into a meaningful and rewarding experience. Our charge was to take a good look at how well we give complete therapeutic treatment not only to patients but also to family and staff. I consider us successful in that we were able to communicate openly to one another our concerns and our accomplishments. As expected, we were not able to come to many conclusions, but we did open several avenues for thought and perhaps future action. The most important result was more awareness and concern for all involved.

INFORMED CONSENT AND PATIENT CARE

Dr. Richie's challenge to take a good look at informed consent set the theme for many intriguing questions such as, "When is a child competent?," "What is the proper perspective when considering a child's consent?," and "Is the consideration even a valid one?" Parents were concerned with their own competence in making decisions under the stress of dealing with a diagnosis of cancer in their children. Usually parents do not have a medical background to help in the decisions; in these discussions the parents said they felt that presentations of alternatives are often biased toward the doctor's preference. This is to be expected as each physician must make his own decision regarding preferred treatment. Parents felt that they must trust their primary physician to guide them. A physician pointed out that so often parents do not have a real opportunity to weigh their decisions because time is critical. A lot of responsibility must be put on the medical profession.

Obviously many of these concerns are unchangable and unanswerable. However, communication between these groups helped us all understand a little better that we are all about the same thing—giving care and concern to one another in a way that will engender both self-respect and mutual respect. A child may not be competent to make his own decisions, but he is worthy of respect and worthy of consideration and explanations within his comprehension.

Mr. Rutherford's presentation sparked many comments on the self-serving or patient-serving nature of the institution and the staff.

Parents expressed concern for the competence of medical students who spend only a month at a time on the ward, during which they must learn many new procedures. They felt they were often in the position of being their child's protectors in determining how much the child can cope with the pain of multiple "sticks," etc. They were supported in the suggestion that they are the best judges of their child's tolerance. It was also brought out that often medical students are the ones who bring about innovations in medicine as well as keeping the staff on its toes by their questions and teaching needs. A staff physician mentioned the difficulty involved with starting IV's on children who no longer have adequate veins. This led to a lively discussion on, "At what point does a physician or nurse admit to not being able to do a procedure?" Parents voiced respect for staff members who are able to say, "I can't do it" or "I don't know."

In considering patient welfare, parents were quick to admit their influence on their children's anxiety levels. They expressed concern about projecting their fears onto the child. Sometimes they felt it best not to participate in areas of treatment that produce trauma in themselves. A technician said that it is much easier for her to do her job if parents are not present. When a social worker countered that it is the child's welfare that must be considered, rather than how much easier the task is, another pointed out that "easier" often includes less anxiety for the child if an anxious parent is not present.

Upon considering another difficult problem existing on 6-West, that of the lack of interpreters for the Spanish-speaking population, many incidents were cited in which poor communication has led to upsets and unfortunate trauma for patients and staff alike. This group of patients and parents is often isolated from activities, such as parent meetings, that would provide the support and information that are such a valuable part of the therapeutic community.

In general, this session was a lively and intriguing one. Many ideas were brought out, and I doubt that anyone left without new concepts to consider. And that is what we were all about.

THE LEADER OF THE TEAM

In the second session of the day, Ms. Chavez and Ms. Buchorn both presented us with much to consider. Ms. Chavez's insight into the nurse's challenges in learning new procedures and providing emotional support to the patient would have provided us with a good basis for discussion. Ms. Buchorn's presentation of the multiple concerns involved with providing a therapeutic community in a pediatric ward would have also done this.

However, such was not to be. As groups will often do, they chose their own direction. There was much laughter and congenial sharing as well as serious consideration given to the subject of who should be "captain of the ship." Also, concern was expressed over how much the patient should know about the diagnosis.

The often amusing discussion on "running the show" was certainly wide in scope. One participant asked, "Why not the head nurse?" (a head nurse in the room vigorously shook her head "no" to this suggestion). Another said that the patient, because he is involved with many professionals at the hospital, is sometimes given contradictory orders. The need for a central person charged with the care of the patient was definitely felt. It led me to fantasize about the possibility of a ward administrator to coordinate all instructions for the patient.

Someone made an analogy between the role of the physician and that of the quarterback on a football team. He felt the need for the medical expert to analyze the positions and direct the play. A chaplain said he experienced tension because he wasn't sure if "I am part of the team. The guy who's the quarterback doesn't ever seem to talk to me about what's going on."

After much discussion about what makes the doctor want to "run the show" and whether he should, a poignant question was asked—would someone define "running the show"? Either someone did and I missed it or the question went unanswered. In any event, a parent made another keen observation. He felt there was a breakdown in communication and he really didn't care who "ran the show." Again I guess we had to ask the question, "What are we all about, anyway?"

Discussion of the knowledge a patient should have about his disease resulted in expressions of vague anxiety by several participants. These expressions came from staff as well as patients and parents. Different staff members verbalized concerns such as, "Can we deal with them like they know everything?," "What are we supposed to keep from the patients?," "What should be told to patients and by whom?" They seemed in need of direct guidance in this area, and I am not sure they received it. Perhaps this could be an area for future consideration in seminar topics.

One parent noted she felt tension in the room at this point. Another stated, "Say what you feel. I'm sorry you feel so apprehensive about talking to patients." A patient expressed hope she would always be told the facts of her disease. Another parent said she felt if the physician did not confront her directly, it was obvious he was uncomfortable with the problem. She also suggested that the support parents need often stems from apprehension in lacking information, and that they often pick their own person to ask for support or information.

Again, I do not feel this issue was resolved, but I do feel we all gained some insight into how much of a problem this really is for everyone. I reiterate, first a guideline is needed.

HOPE AND REALITY

The second day we had the privilege of hearing Dr. van Eys speak on the physical and mental cost to the patient as well as the caregivers (most often identified as staff). He talked of the need to consider that we are now dealing with the cure of the cancer patient. This involves us not only with the medical care of the patient but with his overall mental and emotional development as well.

Mrs. Peterson gave us insight into the dilemmas of the parent dealing with a child stricken with cancer. She acknowledged the need for denial at times, as well as the need for hope. Her presentation left me glad I had come. I was acutely aware of some of the sadness with which we deal. This awareness of beauty and joy as well as sadness and defeat is with us always on 6-West. Perhaps that is why we are all there. The dynamics of life are ever acutely present.

The third discussion group stayed fairly close to the task at hand. Father O'Donnell presented us with a dilemma expressed by Elizabeth Kübler-Ross: the ultimate reality of "child has cancer and may die." How do you balance this reality against hope? And hope for what? Cure? Another day? He felt we have come far enough in taking care of cancer and, as Dr. van Eys expressed it, we now must expect cure, not ultimate death.

Many concerns were expressed, from "How do you maintain normal development?" and "How do you deal with the focus on one child?" to "What is the use of school, anyway?" Parents and staff both supported the view that the most normal home environment is best for the cancer patient. Achieving that ideal is another problem, however, and guidance is often needed. Marital difficulties arise when families are separated for long periods of time. Siblings are often farmed out to relatives and friends. Children in certain stages of the disease must be isolated from groups of people. Future goals for the child are uncertain. Financial stress often exists, especially if the mother has had to give up a necessary job. All are vital concerns and must be dealt with daily by the family.

Obviously it was not within the scope of this symposium to answer all of these concerns. The important objective was to ask the questions and to attempt a start on some of the answers. We were made acutely aware of the humanness of us all through the common concerns expressed and the sharing of our hopes and sorrows. I feel we moved closer to our ideal of teamwork. I also felt very much supported in my task at the hospital. The symposium left me with the knowledge of having accomplished something worthwhile and having learned a great deal about what M. D. Anderson Hospital and its Pediatric Department are all about. Dr. Shaw said when it was all over, "It's kind of sad to say good-bye." I too felt this, as it is difficult to get close to people and their concerns without investing a part of yourself. I feel we were all rewarded for the experience.

CHAPTER 17

A Weekend Together: Impressions

CHARLES R. SHAW

It was a genuine coming together, more successful by far than I had really expected. Almost everybody participated and seemed to get into the spirit of the thing as the weekend progressed. Three two-hour sessions, a couple of dozen people in a room, talking, learning about one another. Coming for what? Not psychotherapy. Unlike a psychotherapy group, with which I am very familiar, they were not coming for help, except in the sense that they wanted to be helped to be better professionals or persons.

My co-leaders for the three sessions were a psychologist (Richard Benton), a psychology student (Terry Rulfs), and a minister (Kenneth Vaux). All were experienced in group work, and hence disinclined to be too directive. Not much silence. The participants, mostly inexperienced in group work, did not feel comfortable with silence. But very little tension either. Somehow they sensed that it was okay to relax. Most of them seemed to feel safe, willing to expose themselves, at least a little. Some, of course, more than others. The less professional people were, not surprisingly, less professional, less restrained, less concerned about role. A physical therapist, a natural, warm woman, spoke of her work with satisfaction, of how it brought her close to the patients: "I lay my hands on them." The patients approach her often as a friend, sometimes with confidences, questions, fears, which they are reluctant to express to the doctors or nurses. She was comfortable in this role, pleased with it, obviously worked spontaneously. But she expressed some reservations and fears about how much to tell the patient. This was a recurrent theme—more about it later.

A preliminary structuring took place at each session as we introduced ourselves to one another. It gave everybody an opportunity to speak out, to be noticed. It seemed to help break the ice, get things started. But I didn't have to work very hard. I remember the whole experience as a pleasantly relaxed one. A bit of initial tension, apprehension, wondering perhaps if the thing would go, but, being experienced, able to stay relaxed and to impart relaxation to the group.

THE NEED TO BE HUMAN

The theme of the workshop, a therapeutic community, delineated in the keynote address by Dr. Vaux, seemed to have gotten across. Permeating the sessions was the feeling that it's alright to be human. The nurses, perhaps more than any other professionals, had difficulty questioning traditional roles, their self-image of the nurse subservient to

153

the doctor. They had difficulty admitting hostility and resentment toward the doctors. The hostility is for private examination and expression, or for gossip. Doctors are authoritarian, and hence engender resentment, particularly those who are incompetent, arrogant, or unfeeling.

The needs of the doctors were aired, and this seemed to generate more feeling than any other single subject. The role of the doctor as leader was considered. Young doctors showed ambivalence about this role, believing that they should not feel superior, but revealing that, in fact, they want and feel they have the right to this role. Doctors were defensive on the subject of how to deal with patients in a mature professional way when they are not yet fully trained and fully confident in their professional status. We discussed whether doctors are trained to assume a professional manner or come to the profession already this way, preselected, so to speak. No specific resolution was reached, but new areas were opened up. The other professionals, as well as parents, expressed some amazement, delight, and sympathy for the problems of the physician, seeing perhaps for the first time the doctor's dilemma, the conflicts among his need to be liked, his need to be an authority, and his fear of not succeeding. We were too polite to come to grips with these issues. I felt a sense of frustration, knowing that we were approaching important material but shying away from it. We laid the groundwork for future sessions, and there should be more, by at least some of the same participants, with perhaps more direction, an opportunity for getting to know one another better and to dig at feelings.

WHAT DO WE TELL THE PATIENTS

What to tell the patients was the overwhelming recurrent question. It came up in every session. But the ways the question was put, and the ways it was dealt with, showed a progress through the meeting. People wrestling with the problem near the end had a much better grasp of it, more insight, more assurance that they could deal with it, than at the beginning. The fear was often expressed that somehow, perhaps by a slip of the tongue, by innocent misphrasing, the patient would be psychologically damaged, dealt some devastating blow. How could this be? We asked those expressing the fear to define, to be specific. There were parents present and one patient, a delightful, wonderfully poised adolescent girl. The message, especially from the girl, was loud and clear: Be honest with us, we need to trust you. On this point, once or twice, I preached a bit. I have heard the same message so often from so many patients. They have told about the early, deceitful, uncertain times, when they know from many cues and signs that they have a serious illness, but are not dealt with openly and know that they are being deceived. They tell of the awful burden and conflict of going along with the act. They tell of the relief when the deceit is over, when somebody, usually the experienced doctor, tells them, "Yes, you have cancer. It is serious. We don't know if you will die, but we will give you the best treatment available."

I think most of the professionals learned this for the first time in the sessions. They seemed satisfied with the concept that they are most effective, most helpful, with the patients and with the parents when they are simply human, themselves, and honest. Rarely, they agreed, was it likely that any of them would be confronted by a patient who knew nothing about his illness, who was ignorant of the fact that he had something serious. Rarely would they be asked directly the question, "What do I have? Is it serious?" The children come to the hospital with all degrees of sophistication, but they have already heard the whispers, seen the anxious and furtive looks between their parents and the doctor. They know that something bad is happening. What do the professionals seeing a child for the first time know about the child's disease that the child does not already know? Sometimes a little more, sometimes a great deal more. But they can be assured that the child will quickly learn.

Another aspect of the same issue: What are the patient's rights? Has he a right to know? The answer of course is yes. It is his body, his disease—he has the right to deal with it the best way he can. He cannot do this in ignorance. The idea of opening up the medical chart to the patient was discussed. To some this seemed almost sacrilege, but the idea was favored by many, especially the more experienced physicians. It may someday, perhaps not too distantly, become a rule.

Does a patient have the right to know that he will die? Of course. The problem here is often *nobody* really knows. We have prognostic impression. But all of us usually retain some hope, even when there is no reason for hope. The parents talked about the need for hope, and about the time when they give up hope. Some seem to want reassurance that this was alright. They received it.

INFORMED CONSENT

More lively discussion. The concept of informed consent was new to many. In the group were a couple of experts, a physician and a member of the human investigation committee. The discussion arose out of Dr. Richie's presentation on clinical research. Again the matter of patients' rights. The patient has the right to decide what will be done with his own body. How can he decide without being fully informed? How can he be fully informed? Does he have the right to decide not only if he will submit to research, but if he will submit to treatment? Put another way, can he refuse treatment? The idea seemed to incense some. If somebody has come to the hospital to see us, they come for help, the best help we can provide. We're the experts. Why should a patient be involved in the decision? As the discussion went on, people moderated their views, grew accustomed to the concept, were again able to question old values. It is not an easy thing to accept. Many of our colleagues, of course, will never accept it, and the course of medical progress will pass them by.

It was pointed out that the concept of informed consent in medicine is but a natural extension of the whole individual rights movement in our society, consistent with recent court decisions on the right of privacy. Some noted that informed consent was being used pragmatically by some professionals to protect themselves, to have a signed document in which the patient has made the decision as to what is to be done with him. This is another of the dilemmas of modern medicine. Someone expressed the hope that the doctrine of informed consent would not impede the progress of medical research. Others noted that it is, in fact, so impeding and will probably continue to do so at an increased rate. There is already a moratorium on fetal research. Much research is either curtailed or abandoned because of problems with obtaining subjects. Supposedly, prisoners can no longer be used for research subjects because they are in a special situation in which they cannot truly give informed consent—there is implied coercion in the fact that they are incarcerated.* More discussion, some expressions of disapproval, talk of the importance of continuing human research, talk of

---

*It is ironic that shortly after this workshop was held, the drive for national protection against "swine flu" began. Prisoners in Texas became the initial test population.

the obligation of every human to help advance medical research. Someone mentioned the position of Dr. Joseph Fletcher, the ethicist, that participation in research is not an infringement on individual liberty but the obligation of every citizen.

AN ATTEMPT AT A CLOSURE

There was no closure really, and I felt the need for one. The time just ran out, and we all got up and wandered into the assembly room for the final address. I remember wanting to say good-bye. I spoke to several others later, and they acknowledged the same feeling. We had sat there together, for the better part of two days, in that special intimacy of a group working together on a common problem. The weather helped: a cold, rainy weekend, good weather for being indoors and being together with others.

Altogether it was a remarkable experience. Jan van Eys conceived it, put it together, carried it through, and I think we all owe him something for that. It took, among other things, some courage. The whole thing could have fallen flat. I know he felt some anxiety about that; I certainly did. But it didn't fall flat. It took off and moved, and a number of people expressed the feeling that they had grown a bit during that weekend together. Warren Rutherford was one of these; I could see that he had, and that he appreciated it. This was, to me, unexpected in one of the management types. You never know.

It was, of course, only a beginning. We must keep working at it, working together, reexamining our roles and our needs and learning how to avoid letting them interfere with our ability to take care of the children's needs. The staff, the ones who work with the children, got glimmerings of what developing a therapeutic community was all about. It will take much more work by all of us. But it's started. I'm optimistic. And I like being a part of it.

CHAPTER 18

Recording the Perceptions of Others

KENNETH VAUX

PATIENTS AND PARENTS,
SPECIALISTS, AND HOME PHYSICIANS

The emphasis of the first group triangulated to three major foci—the patient and his parents, M. D. Anderson, and the home physician—and the interrelationships between these three.

A significant distance exists between the home physician and the other two points. One out-of-town parent described the extreme difficulty of reestablishing a relationship with her child's physician on returning home. The time that elapsed before M. D. Anderson records reached him created a situation in which the mother knew more about her child's cancer than the doctor did. She was put in the position of having to tell the doctor what medication was needed and how often, and she sensed a great deal of hostility resulting from this.

The involvement of the home physician was seen as a necessary component of total care of the patient, yet there are apparently factors that work against this. It is difficult to transmit M. D. Anderson's attitude and philosophy to the home doctor. One M. D. Anderson doctor said, "Some [home] doctors I trust, some I don't. Some patients I keep here for the critical period." Since there is an increasing tendency for patients to return to M. D. Anderson for the treatment of things unrelated to cancer (one child was recently checked for pinworms), the home physician may say, "If they don't trust me with flu, why should I bother with cancer?" "Professional jealousy" was mentioned as a possible explanation for the home physician's hostility but seemed too simplistic in light of the complexity of the illness and treatment, and the intensity of the relationship between parent, patient, and M. D. Anderson. Once a symposium was arranged specifically to involve the private physician, but attendance was extremely poor.

One physician said, "We have so many medical protocols, why couldn't we have communications protocols?" The need for direct communication with the home physician was seen as a necessity for developing a personal relationship between him and M. D. Anderson. The mother who had run afoul of the home physician said it would have helped a great deal to have a brief letter to present to the doctor.

In general we agreed that heightened respect was needed from M. D. Anderson specialists for community physicians. The reciprocal attitude would improve referral mechanisms and generally enhance the patient care which requires the competent ministrations of both doctors.

How do parents feel about M. D. Anderson? Said one mother, "They *gave* our child to us for another year and a half. At home they just said, 'I don't know.' " Another mother responded, "I second that. For us it has been eleven years now, and I have very few gripes." Her son, now twenty-one, said, "I didn't cooperate at first. But now I trust the Anderson doctors, and can't relate to my family doctor." This patient praised M. D. Anderson for always trying to fit its schedule to his. He also stressed telling the child-patient what he has. His own parents tried to shield him, thinking he was too young at ten to handle the information, but by the time he was eleven he had picked up the information and was looking up more in the library.

"A conspiracy of silence" was pointed out to be very debilitating. It was suggested that physicians could develop skills at probing for questions from parents. Although there are many things doctors don't know about cancer, "I don't know" was acknowledged to be an answer in itself. Consistently, though, the plea from patients and parents was, "Tell us what's going on!" One mother asked about the feasibility of a brochure for parents.

Another mother mentioned the growing realization, as her son matured, of the need to allow him to assume responsibility for his own health and recovery. There was also speculation as to whether "we as an institution ever really send a patient home." Some perceived a sort of parental possessiveness on the part of the M. D. Anderson team, and it was observed that everyone referred to "the outside." Is this good? "It has to be," replied one patient, "or we'd lose the sense of being special."

Any one point of the triangle is fraught with some degree of anxiety created by the unknown. For the home physician there are the unknowns of the illness and the treatment. For the patient and the parent there are vast unknowns of prognosis, technology, the nature of the particular cancer, and their own emotional responses. For the M. D. Anderson team there is the awareness of unknowns and limitations of treatment, as well as the unknown of their own emotional responses. A physician from Radiotherapy observed that some nurses are more likely than others to get involved with patients, that the treatment itself tests one's own values and resources. Yet within the area of the triangle a picture develops of a very complex and devastating disease being taken to task by many people in a very cooperative—and very human—way.

DEPERSONALIZATION

"It is amazing," said a chaplain, "that in a hospital where the patient is outnumbered by staff two or three to one, one feels like part of an anonymous mass. We've had to be quite brilliant to depersonalize it; it took a lot of maneuvers. We should explore some of the techniques for making everyone know that their presence is known—that we are cognizant of their needs and that they will be responded to."

The discussion of depersonalization centered on institutionalized frustrations which tend to make both patients and staff feel depersonalized. "There is an institutional indifference to waiting," said one physician. The waiting which clinic patients endure is outrageous and stems from more than one source. Part of it is predictable in that everyone comes to the clinic at once, indicating a pressing need for scheduling. The director of nursing said that this has been done in other areas but hasn't reached Pediatrics yet. Scheduling is done from the standpoint of the individual physician: how many patients he can see, how does he need to be scheduled, how much leeway does he need for emergencies? She also commented that there was a need for someone to expedite problems. One physician pointed out that improvements in the system should begin in Pediatrics because its problems are so much more critical. He observed that, since parents frequently work and have other children, the delays often mean someone is out of work, a child is waiting at home, and a sick child is also waiting.

Another cause of waiting and crowding is parental anxiety and reluctance to leave the floor even for brief periods. "The parents are frightened to death," said one, "that if they do anything against what you want they are not going to get what they need. People will wait and wait to make a complaint because they fear reprisal. We've tried to follow up through the nursing office. This is realistic." Parents of inpatients frequently say, "They tell us to get away, and when we do and come back, they say, 'Where have you been?' or, 'It's about time.'" Several instances of "double messages" were cited. The director of nursing asked how or if this was handled. "It's constantly talked about," was the reply, "but it's not handled in an authoritarian way, because what you're talking about is people's feelings and their own acceptance."

The parents of clinic patients also manifest anxiety and are hesitant to leave the waiting area for fear the doctor will come while they're gone. At one time movies were shown in the auditorium for people who were waiting, but no one would go. They felt they had to show themselves physically. Some parents will not leave no matter what is done to encourage them; others have more spunk and find innovative ways to "beat the system." A suggestion was made that the mothers write a handbook.

The parents emphasized the importance of the person at the clinic desk or unit desk in lessening anxiety. The staff is aware of the need for an "ombudsman," a "high IQ, expediter-type," someone who is not afraid to intercede on behalf of parent and/or patient.

Staff frustrations in part stem from the same source as parent/patient frustration—the crowding due to burgeoning patient load and the transition of some cancers to episodic, long-range illnesses. There is a very high turnover in personnel. The new personnel are not prepared for so many sick children; many are not trained in sick child care at all. Part of the frustration stems from the presence of so many trainees. Currently at M. D. Anderson there are 128 student nurses from three schools with different philosophies. On the other hand, students are often seen to have a clearly positive effect on patients. In any case, future plans for M. D. Anderson include moving more into the role of a teaching facility.

A plea was made for a more multidisciplinary team approach. One physical therapist told of a time a nurse sent a superintelligent, hyperactive four-year-old down to therapy accompanied by a note, "Please keep him for one hour." She said if she had not been familiar with the child's regular habit of tagging behind the doctors and quizzing them about various cases, she would have thought the nurse was crazy. Another therapist said, "I don't know who started it, the yellow sheet up front in Pedi, but if I have a question that really needs answering I always get it answered there. It's a fantastic way of communication and saying thanks."

"I've been interested ever since I've been at Anderson," said a nursing administrator, "in a total patient record—doctor's progress notes, nurse's notes—everybody writes their own thing. Some don't write at all. We really don't have a good vehicle for communication among all the people who are supposed to be focused on the patient."

We discussed the rewards of recognition and stimulation—rewards in terms of multidisciplinary communication and stimulation such as continuing education. There had been covert denials by some of the allied health professional's need for stimulation or education.

Throughout the discussion was woven anticipation of the new facilities, along with awareness that the move will create new problems and call for new mandates. Already mentioned have been the definite scheduling of patients, a total patient record and other forms of staff communication, and a mother's handbook. A need for retraining, for reconditioning, for changing thinking—perhaps a mass meeting for mothers and for staff before the move was also mentioned. "Because people have always done things one way," said one, "doesn't mean it has to continue after the purpose has been served."

HONEST ANSWERS

The last discussion centered around two main themes—answering patients' questions about their illness and society's reaction to the illness once the patients leave the hospital. In a broad sense it can be said that the two are tied together by the concept of human relationships—the relationships of the caregiver to the patient and the patient to society.

One physical therapist said, "We are challenged by parents to be honest as far as our expertise goes, but we have a hard time defining where that begins and ends. Sometimes it's a cop out to say, 'I don't know,' when you really do, but is it acceptable professionally?" An anesthesiologist pointed out that many times he is asked specific questions—about time of surgery, length of stay, hazards—that the surgeon has already answered. He speculated that the repetition of questions is part of the shock, or weighing one answer against another, or simply seeking reassurance.

The physical therapist said one patient insisted she tell him if he was going to die immediately because, if he was, he wanted to write his will. He was convinced she knew when he would die because she had access to his chart. She told him that, since he was eighty years old, perhaps he should write one anyway.

Do you tell children what they have? The answer consistently is, you tell. Someone suggested that the caregivers' hesitancy is rooted in their own discomfort. It was generally agreed that, as in questions about sexuality, children comprehend as much as they are able to handle. Some parents adamantly try to protect their children from information about their illness; this is acknowledged to be a problem, but the children find out one way or another. A critical criterion for "honest answers" seems to be the caregiver's own degree of comfort and ease. One physician said, "I think every answer should be a straight answer, but should contain a hope in it. When we deal with statistics in tumor control, we find out we *don't* know. When I was in medical school, the doctor who set a time limit was a bad doctor."

Another told of a child who kept saying he was going to die, and no one would listen to him. He let them do whatever they had to do to him, but he kept repeating the statement. Finally one day he said to a resident, "I am going to die—now," and he did. A chaplain was asked by a woman, "Am I dying?" When he replied, "I don't know, how do you feel?" she opened up. She wanted to talk to him about the fact that she was dying, about her very deep spiritual experiences. In both instances the patients were asking for someone to listen to them, to relate to them, to not be threatened by their illness, to be at ease with their disease.

Would a child of eight who had been treated for cancer since he was three face the same psychosocial problems that, for instance, a post-open-heart patient would face? One physician said, "Any chronic illness would have the same problems. Cancer has become a chronic illness rather than a predictable outcome. . . . It's very hard to talk about living with a handicap or having somebody living with us who in our eyes is not quite up to par."

A physician commented on the stigma that is placed on cancer as rehabilitated patients go out into their own worlds. Several instances were cited: an amputee who saw a store clerk disinfect the area where she had been shopping, schools assigning visiting teachers when the children are able to go to class, college students not being taken as serious degree candidates.

"I wonder if it is time now," said another physician, "for some type of publication or dissemination of information aimed at the public that would go into more specifics, because cancer has been such a scary word." Several people described the tendency to call by name those cancers which are considered curable, such as Wilms' tumor or Hodgkin's disease. "But I never say 'lymphoma,' " added one doctor.

Are the patients taught ways of handling the societal rejection? They are told to be frank and forthright, but it was generally agreed that ways should be found to teach rehabilitated patients to handle such situations. At one university, students formed a group called "The

Incurables" to make themselves heard by academic authorities. Reference was made to an article, "Deviance Disavowal," which describes processes a person uses to reject society's labeling and rejection. The Leukemia Society Mother's Group was mentioned as a possible vehicle for exploring this area. One volunteer described a pilot program in HISD of health classes in six high schools and said she has been asked to talk to these students about cancer.

The central focus of relationships seemed to be summed up in two closing statements. A physical therapist commented, "Is this any different from teaching physical skills like crutch walking and gait training? Do you accept anything less than maximum? You accept him where he is and then advance forward. There really isn't much difference." "You have to accept people on the therapy team where they are," said a psychiatrist, "and not everybody is equally good. Hopefully we can all get better and not be supercritical of those who aren't."

SECTION VI

Summation

CHAPTER 19

Disease, Suffering, and Hope

KENNETH VAUX

Summarizing and synthesizing the deliberations of such a conference is a formidable challenge. Our discussions ranged from the profound reaches of theodicy, asking why children get sick and die, to mundane issues like why the social psychotherapist has to have her interviews in the ladies' room. We heard the hard realism of business, economics, and management and the lofty visions of the ideal utopia that awaits when we move into the new building. There was much candid and helpful sharing of our perceptions of each other. We had some stereotypes broken, others confirmed. We saw how our own attitudes and actions either contribute to or detract from the therapeutic community. We examined several supposed tensions, dilemmas, conflicts, or dichotomies: biomedical research on or for the patient; the institution as self-serving or patient-serving; the medical, nursing, and social ministries given to vested interest or genuine patient service.

The consensus of our formal presentations and discussion was that there is no essential discrepancy. Ethical criteria and vigorous human protections ensure better research. Just as a lifeguard must first protect his own life before he goes out to save another, so an institution must ensure its own fiscal and structural integrity as it meets the human needs it was designed to serve. Doctors, nurses, therapists, and technicians, each individual on the health team has particular needs, as does each recipient of health care. Love often means hanging in there when we want to run. Love sometimes means letting go. Our respective needs will be met as we honor and serve each other, discovering the truth of the dictum: *Through thee: I am.*

Numerous practical suggestions and recommendations were made and are being considered by administrators and department heads.

A lasting impression was how vital each professional group and special group is in wholistic, comprehensive patient care—the orderlies, attendants, volunteers, desk clerks, lab people, diagnosticians, rehabilitation therapists, pastors, social therapists, nurses, and doctors. Each is indispensable. We must find a better way to give each patient a sense that he is important, that we know he is waiting there, that we care for him. We have two or three employees in the hospital at any time for each patient; it is inexcusable to have patients anguished by the thought, "There is no one here who cares."

All of the insights shared at this conference have been recorded in this book to enable all of us to give each idea careful consideration and implementation. Other hospitals can also review our findings and appropriate them to their practical needs.

Finally, we were reminded in this workshop of the deep reaches of human life that are touched in the hospice of life and living and death and dying in which we are privileged to work. We see courage and hope in the fact of overwhelming challenge. We learn over and over the ancient truth, expressed in the words of Victor Hugo, "The supreme happiness in life is knowing we are loved."

Some of us have personally watched with our own children at death's door; all of us have been near when a young life was received back to the source of all life. All of us have had the beatitude of knowing the meaning of the ancient child's prayer, "If I should die before I wake." We know the bittersweetness, the blended discord and harmony, that life is in its depths. We know the hope mingled with fear while we fight for life in our children; the sorrow mingled with peace, and we render up their lives.

I close with the closing song from Gustav Mahler's *Kindertötenlieder* cycle:

In this weather, in this shower, I would never have sent the children out.
They were dragged out; I was not allowed to say anything against it.
In this weather, in this storm, I would never have let the children go
    out.
I was afraid it would make them ill, but those were vain thoughts.
In this weather, in this awful storm, I would never have let the children
    go out.
I was afraid they would die tomorrow; but there is nothing to do about
    that now.
In this weather, in this awfulness, I would never have sent the children
    out.
They were dragged out: I was not allowed to say anything against it.
In this weather, in this storm, in this shower, they are resting,
Resting as if they were at home with mother. Frightened no more by
    storms,
Watched over by God's hand, they are resting as if they were at home
    with mother.

INDEX